Therapeutic Activities
With the Impaired Elderly

Therapeutic Activities With the Impaired Elderly

Phyllis M. Foster
Editor

The Haworth Press
New York • London

Therapeutic Activities With the Impaired Elderly has also been published as *Activities, Adaptation & Aging,* Volume 8, Numbers 3/4, June 1986.

The Haworth Press, Inc., 28 East 22nd Street, New York, NY 10010-6194
EUROSPAN/Haworth, 3 Henrietta Street, London WC2E 8LU England

Library of Congress Cataloging-in-Publication Data

Therapeutic activities with the impaired elderly.

"Has also been published as Activities, adaptation & aging, volume 8, numbers 3/4, June 1986"—T.p. verso.
Includes bibliographies.
1. Aged—Rehabilitation. 2. Aged—Care and hygiene.
I. Foster, Phyllis M.
RC 953.5.T49 1986 615.8'515'0880565 86-9945
ISBN 0-86656-566-3

Therapeutic Activities
With the Impaired Elderly

Activities, Adaptation & Aging
Volume 8, Numbers 3/4

CONTENTS

**THERAPEUTIC ACTIVITIES WITH THE
IMPAIRED ELDERLY: AN OVERVIEW**

Therapeutic Individual Activities   **1**
    Barbara Szekais

  Activities as Therapy   2
  Categories of Activities   6
  Summary   10

Therapeutic Group Activities   **11**
    Barbara Szekais

  Group Levels   12
  Aspects of Individual Group Members   14
  Categories of Groups   16
  Summary   19

Planning and Leading Activity Groups   **21**
    Barbara Szekais

  Goals and Problems   22
  Leadership   22
  Group Levels   24
  Guidelines for Planning Groups: A 3 Step Process   24
  Summary   28

**"Worth Repeating" Activities and Resources Reference
List for Activities Workers With
the Elderly**   **29**
    Barbara Szekais

Books   29
Publications of Potentials Development for Health
    and Aging Services, Inc. (Buffalo, NY)   33
Publications of The Haworth Press (New York)   34
Journal Articles   34
Journals   35

**Effects of Institutionalization Upon Residents
of Extended Care Facilities**   37
                Judith E. Voelkl

Learned Helplessness   38
Research on Perceived Control   39
Instrumental Passivity   41
Operant Observational Research   42
Implications for Activity Staff   43

**A Protocol for Recreation and Socialization
Programs for the Aged**   47
                Michael J. Salamon

Physical Activities   49
Socialization Groups   51
Board Games   52
Special Events   53
Motivation   53
Additional Considerations   54
Summary   55

**A Humanistic Approach to Old-Old People:
A General Model**   57
                Leonard Babins

**"Worth Repeating" Reality Orientation:
Full Circle**   65
                Geneva Scheihing Folsom

**"Who Did You Used to Be?" The Psychological
Process of Aging's Impact on Institutionalization:
Implications for Activities**   75
                Sally S. Garrigan

"Sign Language Through Discussion" . . . An Innovative Activity   79
> Fred Greenblatt
> Jeffrey Rabinowitz

They Need Us, We Need Them: A Study of the Benefits of Intergenerational Contact   83
> Bonnie B. Lindquist

The Effects of Reminiscing on the Perceived Control and Social Relations of Institutionalized Elderly   95
> Donna E. Schafer
> Forrest J. Berghorn
> David S. Holmes
> Jill S. Quadagno

Method   98
Results   102
Discussion   105
Conclusion   108

The Design and Implementation of Memory Improvement Classes in the Adult Day Care Setting   111
> Evelyn Capuano

Introduction   111
The Decision to Address the Issue   111
Behavioral Objectives   112
The Design and Implementation of Classes   112
Sharing Experiences   113
Providing Memory Tasks   113
The Importance of Imagery   114
Modification for Memory Impaired Individuals   115
Summary   115

The Effects of Pet Facilitative Therapy on Patients and Staff in an Adult Day Care Center   117
> Joanne Damon
> Rita May

Tame Wild Animals 121
Targeted Individuals With Bridget 123
Conclusion 129

**Living With Dying: A Model for Helping Nursing
Home Residents and Staff Deal With Death** **133**
Adele Weiner

**The Relationship Between Nursing Home Residents'
Perceptions of Nursing Staff and Quality of Nursing
Home Care** **143**
Shayna Stein
Margaret W. Linn
Elliott M. Stein

Method 146
Results 148
Discussion 151

**Is Laughter the Best Medicine? A Study of the Effects
of Humor on Perceived Pain and Affect** **157**
Elizabeth R. Adams
Francis A. McGuire

Methodology 160
Results 161
Discussion 173

**The Interface of Activity and Psychopharmacological
Agents** **177**
Leon Hyer
Richard Bagge

Overview of Activity 178
Psychopharmacological Problems 180
Treatment Rules 183
Conclusion 186

**Self Medication as a Form of Self Control in an
Intermediate Care Facility: Preliminary Data** **191**
Michael J. Salamon
Ruth A. Fulger
Salvatore LaVerde

The Present Project 193
Findings to Date 194
Discussion 195

BOOK REVIEWS

Memory Fitness Over 40, by Robin West 199
    Reviewed by Ellen Lederman

Down Memory Lane, by Beckie Karras 200
    Reviewed by Michelle R. Umbaugh

WHAT'S NEW? 203
    Phyllis M. Foster

THERAPEUTIC ACTIVITIES WITH THE IMPAIRED ELDERLY: AN OVERVIEW

Therapeutic Individual Activities

Barbara Szekais

ABSTRACT. Activities can provide a beneficial experience for impaired elderly in a variety of health and social service settings. When coupled with basic knowledge and interdisciplinary effort, activities can be used as an effective therapeutic intervention. Activities which can be used as individual intervention can be organized into at least six categories: crafts, creative expression, personal discovery, environmental involvement, intergenerational involvement, community involvement, and self-directive activities.

Activities form an important intervention approach with the disabled elderly. Impaired elderly people are seen in a variety of health and social service settings, for example Senior Centers, multi-purpose centers, church centers, day care and day health centers, retirement residences, nursing homes, and institutions. A common element among all of

This article was written when the author held the position of Lecturer in the Department of Occupational Therapy at the University of Queensland, St. Lucia, Q 4067, Australia. The author is currently employed in an adult day health center in Seattle, Washington, is a member of the Editorial Board of *Activities, Adaptation & Aging,* and edits the special feature, "Try This . . . ," an activity idea exchange, in that journal. Address inquiries to: 3719 Bagley Ave., North, Seattle, WA 98103.

these settings, which represent a diversity of service foci, is the use of activities. The universality of activities is further testified to by the range of service workers involved in activity programs: activity directors, recreational therapists, occupational therapists, certified occupational therapy aids, social workers, volunteers, nurses, and sometimes even psychologists and physical therapists.

ACTIVITIES AS THERAPY

Some properties of activities are inherently beneficial. Activities represent a positive approach in that they emphasize functional abilities and potential rather than disability. They can be used not only in restoration of function, but also in maintenance and prevention of dysfunction and can be used with a great variety of people and ability levels. Activities stimulate the physical, perceptual, cognitive, and social-emotional abilities of the person (Cynkin, 1979; Hamill & Oliver, 1980).

Activities provide opportunities for active participation, skill acquisition and practise, role performance, realistic appraisal of abilities, and decision making (Fidler, 1981; Johnson, 1981). Because of such opportunities, activities can foster responsibility, meaning, competence, positive self-concept, growth, and change (Cynkin, 1979; Fidler & Fidler, 1978; Huss, 1981; Rogers, 1982).

Activities as individual therapy, however, must be realistic and appropriate. Effective use of activities as therapy depends on (1) knowledge of development and disability, (2) activity analysis, (3) knowledge of the individual elderly person, and (4) awareness of the environment.

Development and Disability

Human development as now understood spans the whole lifetime, not just a certain time during childhood. Adulthood and later adulthood are, just as childhood, a composite of stages, of tasks and challenges for further growth of the individual. The elderly person faces changing life circumstances, both positive and negative, to which he or she must adapt.

Knowledge of normal development and growth is important in understanding these past and present life experiences of the older adult.

Disruption of normal function—or disability—is also necessary to understand. A major disability has definite consequences on a person's functional level, depending on the type of disability and the person's own physical and emotional development. Disabilities impose different kinds of limitations—but also may leave other abilities intact. It is important to understand the nature of particular disabilities, so that expectations of an impaired elderly person are not mistakenly set too high or too low.

In the impaired individual, both the normal developmental process and the disruption of that process determine abilities, limits, and behavior. Knowledge of development and of disability helps in comprehending the individual's present functional level and also the disparity the person may feel between past and present functioning. It can aid in establishing potential directions for change and improvement.

This knowledge is, or should be, part of the training of health care workers such as nurses, physical therapists, occupational therapists, and recreational therapists. Activity workers may or may not have had such training. The point is that *all* those who work with impaired elderly should have access to such information. Staff in-services, continuing education classes, workshops, and community presentations are the places to offer and acquire the information. If such opportunities are not available, the place to start is developing and organizing them. Such knowledge enriches the efforts of activity workers as well as their elderly clients.

Activity Analysis

Activity analysis, the second consideration, is the process of examining the characteristics of individual activities. First, an activity (as normally performed) is broken down into sequential steps. For example, in order to open a door, the steps may be broken down thus: one must (1) stand or sit in front of the door, (2) visually find the knob, (3) bring one arm forward, (4) extend the fingers, (5) grasp the knob, (6) turn the knob, (7) pull, or push, the door open, (8) avoid hitting oneself or others, (9) release the knob. Other factors include having the motivation to open the door and knowing when it is and when it is not appropriate to do so.

Individual Evaluation

Knowledge of the individual elderly person, the third consideration, comes from evaluation. Evaluation provides information concerning the person's background, skills, interests, experiences, strengths, weaknesses, and functional levels. This information is important, because activities are most effective when they are relevant to clients' experience, consistent with their skills and interests, supportive of their strengths, and appropriately adapted to their functional levels.

Evaluation procedures exist to varying in almost all facilities serving the impaired elderly. Formal evaluation exists, for example, as psychiatric evaluations, nursing evaluations, evaluations of gross and fine motor coordination, activities of daily living assessment, and skills and interests inventories. This information, coupled with knowledge of development, disability, and activity analysis, will lead to the activities most suited and beneficial to the individual impaired elderly person.

Evaluation is not mainly formal, however, nor is it static. Each time the impaired elderly person engages in activity, there exists the opportunity for observation and on-going informal assessment. This is a daily process in which all workers have a part and by which all contribute to the general fund of information. The elderly person himself or herself will also contribute information as to the appropriateness, success, or lack of success of an activity; even after the process of thinking through development, disability, characteristics, and individual client information, the elderly person's response to an activity remains the final arbitor of the activity and must be respected.

Once the steps have been clarified, they are looked at in terms of physical, perceptual, cognitive, emotional, and social skills needed to perform them. To open a door, for example, one must have (1) most trunk, arm, and hand muscles of adequate strength, (2) vision sufficient to see the knob, (3) perception sufficient to locate it in space, (4) judgement as to when the door should be opened, (5) recognition of the order in which to perform the steps and the ability to remember them, (6) the desire and the ability to initiate the activity, and, possibly, (7) the ability to greet or deal with someone on the other side.

This is not an exhaustive list for this particular activity, but it amply demonstrates the complexity of even mundane tasks. With the knowledge, or access to the knowledge, of what human physical, perceptual, cognitive, emotional, and social skills are and how they develop, the activity worker can see what skills are required by specific activities and what problems might be anticipated when considering those activities for specific impaired individuals.

In addition, activities need to be examined in terms of materials required, cost and availability of those materials, time involved, space and assistance available, and safety factors. Activities must fit not only clients, but also the facility's physical environment, workload, budget, and philosophy. Activity analysis aids in adapting activities for specific individuals and facilities, and helps to make the experience of the activity positive and successful for all.

The Environment

The last consideration is the environment. The environment is the "silent partner" in the effort to maintain or improve functioning and quality of life. This means making activities directly relevant to the living context. Activities as therapy utilize the person's total environment and offer opportunities for more meaningful involvement in that environment.

Both the physical and social environments of service settings need to provide opportunities for practise of skills and abilities, for example daily living skills, social skills, decision making, and self-expression. Elderly clients need to be encouraged to care for their personal appearance and that of their physical surroundings. They need to be allowed to decide, to the extent possible, the nature of their daily program and how they will participate. They need to see that they have an effect on the quality of their own lives. Individual therapeutic activities cannot remain isolated from the older person's environment, but must be relevant to and practised in that environment.

In a service setting, each individual service worker of whatever discipline can contribute to the above four considerations. Indeed, it is important that activities have the same interdisciplinary approach as other health and social services, as activities can influence all the areas of the elderly person's functioning and thus are a potentially powerful intervention. Interdisciplinary cooperation and communication contribute to the success of that intervention.

CATEGORIES OF ACTIVITIES

A number of activities may be used therapeutically on an individual basis. The following categories of activities are meant to provide a framework relevant to most service settings, to organize conceptually activities that take place in those settings, and to serve as a basis for generating further suggestions for activities. This framework is only one way of viewing activities and is not exhaustive. It does not present activities that most often take place in a group format (e.g., general exercises). Many of the activities suggested here for individuals may in addition take place in a group format; however, individual rather than group activities are the focus of this discussion.

It is possible to distinguish at least six categories of individual activities. The categories include: crafts, creative expression, personal discovery, environmental involvement, intergenerational involvement, community involvement, and self-directive activities.

Crafts

Crafts are possibly the activities in widest use. It is important to remember, however, that there is nothing intrinsically therapeutic about crafts if a person does not want or is not able to do them. Craft activities must be adapted to individual interests and skill levels; with the elderly especially there should be a reason for the craft, a use for it.

There are a number of meaningful reasons for crafts. Some of those reasons include: (1) intrinsic interest and desire; (2) personal or environmental need (e.g., name plates for rooms, place mats for dining tables, writing stationery), (3) reality orientation (e.g., calendars with scheduled events, name tags, seasonal decorations), (4) gifts (e.g., patchwork pillows, bath salts), (5) financial reward (e.g., sale of afghans, tea cozies), (6) beautification (e.g., centerpieces, wall hangings), (7) social interaction (e.g., common quilts), (8) holiday celebrations (e.g., Christmas wreaths, birthday gifts).

Crafts exercise a variety of skills including motor, perceptual, and cognitive abilities. They may serve as a basis for remotivation and resocialization efforts. The purpose of the craft especially and the finished product itself serve as motivating forces, and may serve to enhance self-esteem.

Creative Expression

This in many cases is a logical extension of craft activities. Whereas many crafts involve pre-formed materials and predetermined finished products, creative expression involves more flexibility. Here the older person determines what the final product will be and what materials and procedures are to be used. This usually means the older person is more functionally able, but opportunities for creative expression can be structured for a variety of ability levels, e.g., weavings created by hemiparetic older adults or paintings to which dementia patients have contributed.

Creative expression involves more than just crafts. It can also encompass drama, music, writing, and movement activities. Creative activities foster a high level of individual awareness and initiative in most cases and can contribute to feelings of personal achievement, competence, and self-worth.

Personal Discovery

This area includes activities which can assist in discovering or rediscovering personal history, often in a format which allows sharing with others. This, like creative expression, is a means of self-discovery and may be used with a wide range of impaired elderly people.

The mapping of genealogies is one example of this kind of activity; a life history or an account of an historic or personally significant event are further examples. These may be verbally recounted and discussed, or may be written, tape recorded, drawn, or illustrated with old photographs and memorabilia. If shared with others, they could be part of a life history or reminiscing group, part of a newsletter or booklet, or part of a community program. Personal discovery can facilitate cognitive and emotional functioning. It certainly exercises memory and can help to review and integrate an individual's life experiences and values. It can assist in acceptance of self, add to self-esteem, and promote growth and re-orientation to the present.

Environmental Involvement

Environmental involvement denotes the use of the physical and social environments of a service setting to practise functional skills. This is the concept of milieu therapy: to use the service setting, first to provide continuity with former roles, skills, and values, and second to ensure continuity with formal treatment efforts (Coons, 1978; Laurence & Banks, 1978).

Environmental involvement includes activities that pertain to self-care, care of the physical environment, participation in the social environment, and involvement in decision making processes. Some specific activities might be: choosing one's own clothing and dressing unassisted (although it may take longer), keeping one's own room clean and neat, assisting with actual mealtime tasks such as setting and clearing dishes, watering plants and emptying ashtrays, serving on a resident Council, or deciding upon one's own recreational schedule. The range of activities is determined by the particular service setting's environment.

These activities need to be graded to individual functional levels and require some assistance and judgement on the part of service workers. However, these activities should be used as much as possible, as it is in large part the environment that gives meaning, value and reward to any individual's activities.

Intergenerational Involvement

Service settings for the elderly generally tend to isolate the older person from other age groups. To a degree, this is appropriate, functional, and may be heartily desired by the older person. Yet very few elderly desire total segregation, and there is much to be gained from activities which include younger people.

Some possibilities in this area include: volunteer and "Friendly Neighbor" programs which involve middle aged adults from families, service organizations, and the surrounding community; educational exchanges with high schools and youth organizations; and foster grandparent programs in elementary schools and children's day care centers. These programs can be run on an on-going basis or may be a single event, such as a holiday program.

The actual activities depend upon the organizations and the potential that exist in the community surrounding the service setting. Such activities with other generations can encourage skill practise and provide an opportunity for appropriate role performance. They also afford opportunities for positive and satisfying social interaction and emotional relationships.

Self-Direction

In this category of activities, the older person is more involved in decision making and takes more responsibility for events and activities in the environment. This type of activity usually demands a higher level of functioning, but again, opportunities can be created and adapted to individual skill levels.

A service setting can include its elderly in a variety of ways. For example, individuals can be consulted for input or a "vote" when activities or procedures are being established or revised; many settings have a Council as a forum for discussion, input, suggestions, and advice to staff. This author was involved in three self-directive activities. In the first, impaired elderly were assisted to attain independent management of the setting's Bingo games, including setting up the games, calling, cleaning up, setting schedules, and making rules. In another instance, two elderly female stroke victims became leaders of a knitting and crocheting group for children from an after-school day care center. In the last case, a woman with a diagnosis of depression was assisted in using her strong faith and religious background to run two sessions of a Bible group for other disabled elderly.

Discretion and caution need to be exercised in using such activities. The service workers in a setting are responsible for structuring and pacing such activities so that performance remains a positive experience for all concerned. When used judiciously, however, such activities can be tremendously satisfying and growth producing, as the elderly individuals see themselves as contributors, leaders, and decision makers in their own lives.

SUMMARY

Activities have characteristics which make them a major intervention approach in working with the impaired elderly and are used in a variety of service settings. Certain background knowledge on the part of the service worker, such as knowledge of development and disability, activity analysis, evaluation information, and the role of the environment, helps to make activities as intervention more effective. The use of activities, like any other intervention, benefits from interdisciplinary cooperation and communication. In considering activities to use, the service worker can use the following categories as an organizing framework and a basis for generating new ideas: crafts, creative expression, environmental involvement, intergenerational involvement, community involvement, and self-directive activities.

REFERENCES

Coons, D.H. Milieu therapy. In W. Reichel (Ed.), *Clinical Aspects of Aging.* Baltimore: Williams & Wilkins, 1978.

Cynkin, S. *Occupational Therapy: Toward Health through Activities.* Boston: Little & Brown, 1979.

Fidler, G.S. From crafts to competence. *American Journal of Occupational Therapy,* 1981, 35(9), 567–573.

Fidler, G.S. & Fidler, J.W. Doing and becoming: Purposeful action and self-actualization. *American Journal of Occupational Therapy,* 1978, 32(5), 305–310.

Hamill, C.M. & Oliver, R.C. *Therapeutic Activities for the Handicapped Elderly.* Rockville, MD: Aspen, 1980.

Huss, A.J. From kinesiology to adaptation. *American Journal of Occupational Therapy,* 1981, 35(9), 574–580.

Johnson, J. Old values—new directions: Competence, adaptation, integration. *American Journal of Occupational Therapy,* 1981, 35(9), 589–598.

Laurence, M.K. & Banks, S.I. Milieu therapy and the elderly: A role for the occupational therapist. *Canadian Journal of Occupational Therapy,* 1978, 45(4), 171–173.

Rogers, J. The spirit of independence: The evolution of a philosophy. *American Journal of Occupational Therapy,* 1982, 36(11), 709–715.

Therapeutic Group Activities

Barbara Szekais

ABSTRACT. Groups are being used more frequently as an intervention approach in health and social service settings for the impaired elderly. As part of an on-going activities program, groups can offer a therapeutic experience to a large number of individuals. This discussion presents reasons for using a group format for activities, essential knowledge and skills of the group leader, and six categories of groups that can be used in a variety of service settings.

In planning activities for the impaired elderly, use of a group format is an option which should be considered. Groups have been adapted for intervention with a variety of ages and disabilities, and are being used successfully with the impaired elderly (Berger & Berger, 1972; Burnside, 1978; Harris, 1979; Jones & Clark, 1981; Kartman, 1979; Maizler, Solomon, & Ronch, 1979; Stabler, 1981).

There are a number of reasons for using a group approach to activities. Groups are a natural experience; almost all learning, development, and change occurs within a group context from the time of birth. Groups are a means for satisfying survival needs, social needs, educational needs, and growth needs (Sweeney, 1975). Groups provide greater opportunities for skill practice, feedback, and support. Groups allow greater numbers of people to be involved in a therapeutic situation and at the same time allow greater independence for group members.

Groups may be used for brief interventions or may be part of an on-going activities program (Storandt, 1978). It is with the latter that this discussion is concerned. Within an activities program, groups can serve a number of different purposes: to reorient and resocialize; to develop support and a sense of belonging; to provide education and skill mastery; to encourage self-expression; to develop responsibility and decision making; and to foster cooperation and task achievement (Burnside, 1970; Mayadas & Hink, 1974; Shere, 1971).

In one survey in a long-term care setting, impaired older people themselves listed reasons for group attendance (Maizler, Solomon, & Ronch, 1979). Their reasons included: opportunity to discuss concerns and feelings; increased privacy and confidentiality; meaningful relationships; a feeling of continuity and of belonging to a cohesive body; social contact; and support for group members.

In using groups as part of an activities program, group leaders and activities personnel will find certain background information helpful in making their groups more successful. This information includes knowledge of group dynamics and leadership skills, understanding of group levels, aspects of the individual members, and some possible categories of groups. Group dynamics and leadership skills are regrettably beyond the scope of this discussion; the reader will find an excellent discussion of dynamics and leadership in Burnside (1984), Levine (1979), Marram (1973), Merrill (1967 & 1974), and Yalom (1975). This paper will discuss group levels, aspects of the elderly group members, and some categories of groups, with examples.

GROUP LEVELS

It is essential that a group leader have a basic understanding of group levels. The term "group level" refers to the skills required in a group situation, either by a task and/or by social interactions. All groups present a demand situation. If the task or social demands placed upon a person are too difficult, that person may feel frustrated, discouraged, angry, or frightened, and most probably will not return to the group. Conversely, if the demands are too low, the person may feel bored, unchallenged, irritated, or frustrated, and again will probably not return to the group. An appropriate match between individual and group depends first on understanding the level at which a group will function. With many activities, the group format can be successfully adapted to a range of group levels.

A brief outline of four group levels will be presented here. This framework is based on a five-level model proposed by Mosey (1970); in working with the impaired elderly, this author found group functioning not quite as differentiated.

The first level is the parallel group. In a parallel group, members are in close physical proximity, and each member works on his or her individual task or just watches. There may be only minimal interaction or sharing of activity, if any. This is the least threatening type of group, the least demanding, and may be used for purposes of resocialization and reorientation. Some typical groups structured for this level may include, for example, movie and travel slide groups, singing and music groups, outings and field trips, Bingo, and simpler crafts.

The second level is the project group. Here group members may engage in a short-term activity that requires some cooperation and interaction. More demands are placed on the members in that some participation and social exchange are required. Examples of a project group may be crafts, cooking, exercise, structured reality orientation, Bible study and spiritual worship, some games such as cards or Scrabble, and general discussion and information groups such as current events or reminiscing.

The third level is the cooperative group. In this group, members engage in a longer term activity in which many aspects are shared. In this group there are common interests and concerns, and a sense of mutuality and belonging. Again, more demands are placed on members, as more participation is required and some self-disclosure is necessary. Groups functioning at this level may include, for example, assertiveness training, communication skills, diet and health, newsletter, a men's or women's discussion group, or living skills retraining groups.

The highest level group is the mature group, where members engage in long-term activities of mutual interest and concern. There may be a common diagnosis or problem in addition. There is an increased sense of belonging and responsibility, and leadership may at times be shared among the members. Trust develops between members which may carry over to situations outside the group. Increased participation and self-disclosure are the norms in this highest level group. Some examples may be life review, psychotherapy, interpretive art, resident/client councils, social clubs, stroke (and other disability) discussion and self-help groups, and family groups.

It is evident that these group levels represent a continuum of increasingly difficult physical, cognitive, and social-emotional skills. If appropriately placed, an impaired elderly person can exercise these skills and progress to higher levels or avoid unnecessary deterioration.

ASPECTS OF INDIVIDUAL GROUP MEMBERS

The impaired elderly individual is the second half of the person-group match. To appropriately place individuals in a specific group situation, certain information concerning the individuals must be available. This information is usually obtained through a formal or informal evaluation process which considers at least three basic areas of functional skills, i.e. physical, cognitive, and socio-emotional skills (Lago & Hoffman, 1977–78).

Physical function concerns, for example, ambulation and mobility, continence, gross and fine motor skills, endurance, and sensory function. Cognitive function includes such aspects as alertness, attention span, memory, verbal ability, learning capacity, and judgement. Social-emotional function takes into account factors such as passivity-activity, socialization habits, communication skills, motivation, and affect. These and other functional skills may be included in an evaluation process.

Evaluation, as discussed in the previous article, usually exists as psychiatric assessments, nursing evaluations, gross and fine motor coordination evaluations, activities of daily living assessments, sensory-perceptual evaluations, and/or interest and skill inventories, for example. Formal evaluation is usually performed by trained health care professionals, such as doctors, psychiatrists, nurses, occupational therapists, recreational therapists. This information is used and shared by all health care workers however, just as all health care workers contribute to the process of on-going informal assessment and observation.

While the above list of skills to be evaluated is not exhaustive, it is already apparent that a number of problems might arise in a group situation. A group leader may be faced with such problems as poor endurance, distractibility, incontinence, sensory deficits, monopolizing verbal behavior, silence, bizarre behavior, apathy, or anxiety (Lago & Hoffman, 1977–78; Yalom & Terrazas, 1968). The group as well as the leader must be ready and able to accommodate these problems. The group leader needs to be aware of the members' skill levels before accepting them into the group and to be able either to change group membership to fit the group level or change the group level to fit membership, as necessary.

For example, the parallel group situation is probably the most appropriate for an individual with moderate to severely impaired memory, impaired concentration and attention span, marked anxiety, inappropriate social behaviors, or very limited physical ability, among other impairments. In the parallel group, maladaptive socio-emotional behaviors will be least disruptive and the learning of more adaptive behaviors can begin. Individuals with severely limited physical abilities can find assistance geared to their needs and an opportunity to adjust to being with others in a positive, supportive situation. Individuals with moderate to severely impaired cognitive abilities can also participate in activities appropriate to their skill levels and receive assistance appropriate to their needs.

Because such problems are a reality in groups with the impaired elderly, the group leader may use a number of less traditional group approaches. These approaches include: (1) less confrontation and more support for group members; (2) more frequent use of structure and directive leadership; (3) smaller numbers of members (5–8); (4) less material with less complexity per group session; (5) slower pace and presentation of material; (6) increased cues, feedback, and positive reinforcement; (7) more repetition and practise; (8) shorter sessions; (9) structured physical environment to enhance sensory function and social interaction; and (10) opportunities to apply the material in the environment outside the group sessions.

The higher the individual's physical, social-emotional, and cognitive skill level, the higher the group level in which that individual will be able to function and benefit. Individuals may initially start at a high group level, or begin at a lower level and progress upward, or stay at lower group levels, depending on their abilities. Group level should match an individual's static or changing functional skills.

Each group is unique, of course, and will present its own special configuration of members' strengths and weaknesses. But the better the match between group and individual, the better able will be the group to facilitate strengths and accommodate weaknesses.

CATEGORIES OF GROUPS

A number of groups can be adapted for use with a variety of impairments and functional levels. Just as a range of individual activities needs to be available, a range of group activities and group levels needs to be present in order to address the various needs of a setting's elderly individuals.

The groups to be suggested here are organized into six general categories. Groups in each category can be structured to operate at different group levels. The categories include: social and recreational groups, education groups, skill training groups, psychosocial therapy groups, self-help groups, spiritual groups, and family groups.

Social and Recreational Groups

These groups cover a wide range of social and recreational activities and can serve three different purposes. The first purpose is resocialization for those at lower levels of functioning; the second purpose is recreation and socialization for those more able to participate and interact; and the third is creative expression and interaction for those at higher levels of function. These purposes correspond, respectively, to the first three group levels, i.e., parallel, project, and cooperative groups.

Possible activity groups may be crafts, outings, adapted sports and games, drama, movies and slides, group reading and humor, fashion shows, holiday activities, poem or song writing, singing, and intergenerational activities.

Education Groups

Education groups can have two different aims in encouraging learning. One aim is to simply disseminate or make available information; this does not require much participation or interaction. The second aim does require higher levels of participation and interaction in that it involves discussion and other processing (e.g., exercises and "homework") of the information presented. It is evident that these two aims represent two levels of difficulty corresponding to group levels two (project group) and three (cooperative group). Examples of education groups include history, reminiscing, music appreciation, Senior health education, and current events.

Skill Training Groups

Groups in this category address a variety of daily living skills and can have two purposes. The first is skill maintenance, i.e., practise of skills already acquired but impaired or not recently used. The second purpose is skill acquisition, which involves learning and practising skills not part of the individuals' behavior. These two purposes correspond respectively to group levels two (project group) and three (cooperative group).

Groups which may be found in this category are physical self-care skills (e.g., grooming or dressing), medication management, exercises, crafts, assertiveness training, diet and nutrition, stress management, communication skills, or use of community resources (public transport, recreation, etc.). Such groups as reality orientation and cognitive retraining would fall into the skill maintenance category, but obviously would have to be structured for impaired elderly at lower functional levels.

Psychosocial Therapy Groups

This category of group includes, again, two possible purposes. The first purpose served is that of discussion/ventilation and support for members, and the second purpose is more intensive self-examination involving more self-disclosure, confrontation, and willingness to change. These two purposes represent, respectively, groups levels three (cooperative group) and four (mature group). Both usually involve more verbal activity, although such techniques as painting or collage, role-playing, and movement may also be used. It is very important with this type of group that the group leader have training in group process, dynamics, and leadership, as these special skills are most necessary to the group's success.

In this category might be found such groups as stroke discussion, life review, men's or women's discussion groups, self-esteem and self-awareness, family groups (without family members present), interpretive art, movement therapy, psychodrama, and transition groups (i.e., transition to different living or treatment settings.)

Self-Help Groups

This type of group most often requires higher levels of independence, initiative, and functional ability in group members, in spite of whatever impairments exist. As such, this group corresponds to group levels four (mature group) and sometimes three (cooperative group). Some typical self-help groups include stroke (and other disability) self-help groups, widow support groups, political action groups, community service groups, resident/client councils, resident/client volunteers (who take care of a setting's physical environment), and on-going resident/client newsletters or other publications. Themes and material for these groups often come from the elderly group members themselves and are often quite specific to individual service settings.

Spiritual Groups

This type of group seeks to respond to a deep need for many elderly, that of spiritual worship and sharing of spiritual beliefs and values. Such groups can be structured to function at a single group level or to include individuals at various functional skill levels. Such groups may have as purposes the activity of worship, education, support, and self-examination. Spiritual groups might include periodic worship services, religious discussion, hymn singing, world religions education groups, and intergenerational religious activities.

Family Involvement Groups

These groups attempt to directly involve family members from outside the service setting and may serve a number of purposes, for example socialization and recreation, education, skill acquisition, psychosocial therapy, and self-help. Family members may be in a group with their elderly relative or may be in a group by themselves. Examples of family involvement groups include outings with family members, open house or holiday activities, disability information and discussion groups, training in managing the impaired older relative, stress management, support and self-help groups such as an Alzheimer's or Parkinson's spouse support group, and family advisory boards.

SUMMARY

Groups can be an effective intervention approach for improvement of skills and quality of life for impaired elderly individuals. Successful use of groups depends on the leader's knowledge of group dynamics and leadership skills, understanding of group levels, awareness of individual members' functional levels, and awareness of the different types of groups. Groups are flexible and can be adapted to varying functional levels of individuals and to various service settings. It is evident that the range of groups can be as wide as the range of needs in a service setting.

REFERENCES

Berger, M.M. & Berger, L.F. Psychogeriatric group approaches. In C.J. Sager & H.S. Kaplan (Eds.), *Progress in Group and Family Therapy.* New York: Brunner/Mazel, 1972.

Burnside, I.M. Group work with the aged: Selected literature. *Gerontologist,* 1970, 10(3), 241–246.

Burnside, I. *Working with the Elderly: Group Processes and Techniques* (2nd Ed.). Monterey, CA: Wadsworth Health Sciences, 1984.

Harris, P.B. Being old: A confrontation group with nursing home residents. *Health and Social Work,* 1979, 4(1), 152–166.

Jones, G.M. & Clark, P. Multidisciplinary group work on a psychogeriatric ward. *British Journal of Occupational Therapy,* 1981, 44(8), 253–254.

Kartman, L.L. Therapeutic group activities in nursing homes. *Health and Social Work,* 1979, 4(2), 135–144.

Lago, D. & Hoffman, S. Structured group interaction: An intervention strategy for the continued development of elderly populations. *International Journal of Aging and Human Development,* 1977–78, 8(4), 311–324.

Levine, B. *Group Psychotherapy: Practice and Development.* Englewood Cliffs, NJ: Prentice-Hall, 1979.

Maizler, J.S., Solomon, J.R., & Ronch, J.L. Group therapy with nursing home residents: A survey. *Health and Social Work,* 1979, 4(1), 211–218.

Marram, G.D. *The Group Approach in Nursing Practice.* St. Louis: C.V. Mosby, 1973.

Mayadas, N.S. & Hink, D.L. Group work with the aging. *The Gerontologist,* 1974, 14, 440–445.

Merrill, T. *Activities for the Aged and Infirm.* Springfield, IL: C.C. Thomas, 1967.

Merrill, T. *Discussion Topics for Oldsters in Nursing Homes.* Springfield, IL: C.C. Thomas, 1974.

Mosey, A.C. *Three Frames of Reference for Mental Health.* Thorofare, NJ: Chas. B. Slack, 1970.

Shere, E.S. Group work with the very old. In R. Kastenbaum (Ed.), *New Thoughts on Old Age.* New York: Springer, 1971.

Stabler, N. The use of groups in day centers for older adults. *Social Work with Groups,* 1981, 4(3/4), 49–58.

Storandt, M. Other approaches to therapy. In M. Storandt, I.C. Siegler, & M.F. Elias (Eds.), *The Clinical Psychology of Aging.* New York: Plenum Press, 1978.

Sweeney, B. Learning groups: Survival level, growth level. *Journal of Nursing Education,* 1975, 14(3), 20–25.

Yalom, I.D. *The Theory and Practice of Group Psychotherapy* (2nd Ed.). New York: Basic Books, 1975.

Yalom, I. & Terrazas, F. Group therapy for psychotic elderly patients. *American Journal of Nursing,* 1968, 68, 1690–1694.

Planning and Leading
Activity Groups

Barbara Szekais

ABSTRACT. Use of activity groups with the impaired elderly can be of potential benefit in an on-going activities program. This article presents some practical information concerning group goals, possible problems, leadership approaches, and planning guidelines for use in implementing activity groups with the impaired elderly.

Participation and membership in a group can be a satisfying and growth-producing experience for many individuals, including the impaired elderly. Whatever the designated purpose—recreational, social, or therapeutic—all groups have the potential for facilitating growth and change in their members. In this sense, all groups can be said to be therapeutic.

Groups can fulfill this potential for growth and change if those who lead them have a basic understanding of some theoretical and practical aspects of groups. This discussion will touch upon some of the theoretical aspects and will concentrate on practical considerations for planning and leading activity groups with the impaired elderly.

Some basic tenets of using groups in an activities program are well-known. Groups should always be based on the interests, skills, and needs of the potential group members. Groups should present a variety of situations: physical movement and verbal interaction, stimulating and relaxing, open (i.e., fluctuating membership) and closed (i.e., fixed membership), large and small, and homogeneous and heterogeneous skills levels of members. In addition to these basic tenets, other aspects of groups deserve attention: goals and potential problems, leadership approaches, groups levels, and planning procedures.

GOALS AND PROBLEMS

The group leader needs to be aware of the basic goals of groups and of the possible obstacles that may be encountered. Goals for groups are various: to maintain or regain optimal levels of physical, social, cognitive, and emotional functioning; to socialize and be part of a supportive community; to feel needed and useful; to have responsibility; to gain respect and approval; and to enjoy oneself and be creative. A successful group can achieve one or a number of these goals.

In attempting to attain these goals in a group for impaired elderly, a number of problems may present themselves. The first type of problem relates to the diversity of physical abilities. Each individual will exhibit decreased ability in one or various areas of functioning. As each individual is different, there may be a variety of disabilities and skill levels within a single group. Often, because of this variety of disabilities, there is a need for assistance in leading the group, and this assistance may not be available or planned for.

Second, group members' attitudes can present problems. The members most probably recognize that they do indeed have deficits, and they may not want to risk exposure of those deficits to others or even to themselves. This awareness of decreased functioning may decrease motivation to participate. In addition, the elderly group members may not have developed leisure interests or any desire or respect for leisure pursuits.

The last type of problem is posed by the group leader's attitudes and abilities. The leader may not know the activity or topic of a group well enough to present the material in an enthusiastic or stimulating manner. The leader may have limited energy to motivate the group, and he or she may possibly react negatively to some of the attitudes of group members discussed above.

LEADERSHIP

There are a number of guidelines and suggestions for effectively leading a group and dealing with problems such as listed above. The first guideline is to be aware of these possible problems. Some of them can be eliminated by prior planning; some cannot be eliminated, but awareness and acceptance of them by the group leader can create a more accepting, less anxious atmosphere in the group.

More specific guidelines concern the leader, the members, and the activity. Concerning the leader: (1) the leader will most likely need to play a strong leadership role, creating both the expectation and the opportunity for participation; (2) the leader needs to be aware of group dynamics and group levels; (3) the leader needs to be enthusiastic, as he or she is a role model and thus a major force in creating interest and enthusiasm; (4) the leader needs to know and respect his or her own attitudes, skills, and limits; (5) and finally the leader should use tact in running the group.

Concerning the members: (1) the leader should solicit the interests and desires of the members and *listen* to them in all phases of planning and execution of the group; and (2) the leader needs to know the members' strengths, limitations, and problems.

Concerning the activity: (1) the leader must know the activity or topic—the group is not the place to be trying it for the first time; here, experience in individual activities, activity analysis, and adaptation will be very helpful; (2) the activity or topic must fit the group level and the individual members' functional skills (e.g., assertiveness training would not be appropriate for a group of clients/residents with Alzheimer's disease nor would crocheting be appropriate for those with Parkinsonian fine motor tremor); (3) the leader must be sure the environment is conducive to the group's functioning, i.e., there is sufficient lighting, seating, privacy, and/or materials, etc; (4) the leader needs to make liberal use of explanation, demonstration, cues, feedback, and positive reinforcement as aids to learning; and (5) the leader must arrange for enough assistance, if required, or limit the number of group members.

In addition to these considerations, some less traditional group approaches were discussed in the previous article. The reader is referred to that discussion for further suggestions.

Motivating is a special part of leading a group, and certainly not the easiest. To help develop motivation for group attendance and participation, the leader may try a number of approaches. The leader needs to make contact with the potential members first, to seek them out and solicit their interests and presence in the group. The leader needs to go slowly, at the pace of the potential elderly member, and to not overwhelm or insist. The leader needs to be respectful and to inspire respect and interest. The more closely a leader matches an activity or topic to the potential member's needs, interests, and abilities, the more willing they will be to participate. These are just a few suggestions for increasing motivation. More extensive discussion and suggestions can be found in Merrill (1967 & 1974).

GROUP LEVELS

Awareness of group levels is essential in order to match the functional level and skills of the impaired older person with the demands of particular group situations. Groups can be structured to require more or less complex skills, and care must be taken that individuals are not placed in group situations where too much or too little is demanded of them. Based on a model proposed by Mosey (1970), four group levels can be distinguished among groups for the impaired elderly: parallel groups, project groups, cooperative groups, and mature groups. These groups represent respectively a hierarchy of increasing demand situations. Group levels and examples are discussed in more detail in the previous article, and the reader is referred to that discussion.

GUIDELINES FOR PLANNING GROUPS:
A 3 STEP PROCESS

Step 1

A successful group needs not only background information, as stated above, but also some prior planning before the group starts. The first step is to make sure the group topic or activity is relevant to the intended group members. This means knowing the population, being familiar with the needs, abilities, interests, and limitations of the potential elderly group members.

Another part of step one is to know the service setting and

what it can offer in terms of space, equipment, materials, financial resources, and administrative support. Some groups require privacy, some require materials, some need special equipment, etc. The environment should be able to provide what is necessary for the success of the group.

It should be remembered that both clients and environment change over time. Having determined needs, interests, and resources once may not be enough; the formal or informal process of assessing the elderly population and the service setting is on-going.

Step 2

Once having selected a need or an interest as the basis of a group, the second step is to plan the group as a whole. Here a number of questions must be answered: (1) The goal(s) of the group must first be determined. General goals stated at the beginning of this discussion were goals applicable to almost any group. Now, the leader must decide the goal of the specific group. For example, the goal of an assertiveness group may be to show assertive behavior more often, or the goal of a Metro group may be to learn to use public transportation, or the goal of a craft group may be to complete a project using a certain art medium. (2) After the goal, specific objectives need to be determined. These are short-term aims that help in reaching the longer term goal. Objectives may turn out to be the topic or activity for each individual group session. An objective for increasing assertive behavior may be to learn how to say no when approached for money or a cigarette; an objective for using public transportation may be learning to read bus schedules; an objective for completing a craft project may be sanding wood in preparation for decoupage.

A corollary to setting goals and objectives is (3) deciding the total number of group sessions and their schedule. A group may run for 10 weeks with two sessions per week, or for six months with one session per week, etc. Different activities and different impairments will result in varying schedules. The important point is to define the beginning and the end of the group. This kind of definition helps to make planning more definite, helps to establish the idea of forward movement during the life of the group, and helps to prevent burn-out of the group leader and members.

At this point an outline can be made of the group, i.e., the overall goal, the objectives, and the time frame. For example: Craft group, 4 weeks, 1 session per week; goal: to produce with minimum level of assistance a patchwork pillow; session 1—objective: select and cut material according to pattern; session 2—objective: begin stitching pattern pieces together by hand or machine; session 3—objective: finish stitching pieces together; session 4—objective: stuff and finish off pillows. A second example: Reading group, 10 weeks, 2 sessions per week; goal: to select, read, and discuss as a group a book of mutual interest; session 1—objective: become acquainted with each other, compile list of interests and possible reading material; session 2—objective: decide upon a book, compile list of willing readers, begin to read; sessions 3–8—objective: read and discuss book and members' comments; sessions 9–10—objective: review book and all important points from discussions; discuss what group members have enjoyed, learned, and gained.

Higher level groups can be planned in the same way. For example: Depression group, 12 weeks, 2 sessions per week; goals (tentative): to gain understanding of causes of depression, to develop trust and support, to improve affect; session 1—objective: become acquainted, establish group goals and rules, discuss being together as a group; session 2—objective: discuss loss as a cause of depression, list losses of the elderly using group members' experiences as illustration, etc. With higher level groups, more flexibility and room for members' input should be allowed. Even with the higher level groups, however, some structure is necessary for the group to progress toward its goals.

Having outlined goals, objectives, and time frames, the group leader then needs to consider the following: (4) the group level, which may already be indicated by the nature of the goals and objectives; (5) minimum and maximum size of the group; (6) number of leaders and/or assistants; (7) length of each session; (8) criteria for selection of members and exclusion (if appropriate) of others; (9) admission of new members—an "open" group will accept new members after the group has started into its schedule, and a "closed" group does not accept new members (e.g., a psychosocial therapy group); (10) rules or codes of behavior, e.g., regarding attendance, punctuality, talking; (11) the physical environment necessary or available; and (12) materials and/or equipment necessary or available.

In lower level groups, the group leader(s) will make most of these decisions. In higher level groups, inclusion of members' ideas and the process of group decision making should be an integral part of the group.

Step 3

The third step is to plan each individual session. The nature of the individual session will be determined in large part by the decisions made in step two, i.e., group level, goals and objectives, length, equipment, etc., and by the leader's knowledge of the group members reached in step one. The group leader will still need to decide upon the format for each session: will it be tightly or loosely structured? Will there be focused topics and exercises or free activity and discussion? Will there be physical activity or verbal discussion or both? Will participation be required or just attendance?

The activity or topic of each session must be determined if it is not already stated as an objective. For lower level groups, the leader will also have to decide upon the specific content of the session and its presentation. In higher level groups, the content may be determined with more assistance from the group members during the session itself. However, even with higher level groups, the leader needs to be prepared for that inevitable session which just doesn't "move" and where the leader then must supply much of the structure and content.

It may be of assistance to the group leader to perform, formally or informally, a pre- and post-session analysis. This does not have to be a complicated task; even brief notes can help the leader prepare for the unpreparable and to summarize what actually happened in a session (for example, see Burnside, 1971).

The pre-session analysis can be a simple listing of: session objective, intended activity or topic, what might go wrong, how to respond, and possible alternative activities. This simple strategy helps the group leader to respond more quickly to unplanned events by anticipating them in advance or at least anticipating the possibility of unplanned events. The post-session analysis might involve brief notations concerning: actual activity or topic, group members present, what transpired during the session, whether the objective was achieved and why. Having a record of what actually happened in group sessions is valuable in spotting changes, progress, and patterns. It also serves as an aid to planning for individual members and for future groups.

SUMMARY

Groups can provide a satisfying and rewarding experience for the impaired elderly, and groups can enrich and enlarge an on-going activities program in a health or social service setting. Effective use of groups requires a certain amount of knowledge on the part of the group leader and a willingness to do some prior preparation and planning. This investment can be well worth the effort, both for the group members and for the leader.

SUGGESTED READING

Burnside, I.M. *Working with the Elderly: Group Processes and Techniques* (2nd Ed.). Monterey, CA: Wadsworth Health Sciences, 1984.
Marram, G.D. *The Group Approach in Nursing Practice.* St. Louis: C.V. Mosby, 1973.
Yalom, I.D. *The Theory and Practice of Group Psychotherapy* (2nd Ed.). New York: Basic Books, 1975.

REFERENCES

Burnside, I.M. Long-term group work with the hospitalized aged. *Gerontologist,* 1971, 11, 213–218.
Merrill, T. *Activities for the Aged and Infirm.* Springfield, IL: C.C. Thomas, 1967.
Merrill, T. *Discussion Topics for Oldsters in Nursing Homes.* Springfield, IL: C.C. Thomas, 1974.
Mosey, A.C. *Three Frames of Reference for Mental Health.* Thorofare, NJ: Chas. B. Slack, 1970.

"Worth Repeating" Activities and Resources Reference List for Activities Workers With the Elderly

Barbara Szekais

The following is an extensive, but by no means definitive, list of written materials which may serve as sources of ideas for activities and activity planning. The focus of these references is practical, not theoretical; some theroretical material which lends itself to practical application has been included. Some references in this list pertain to individual activities, some to group activities; some references list specific activities and projects, while some may serve as topics for discussion and reflection; some of these books are concerned with planning, and some with doing; some books are very recent and some very old; some of the references contain ideas which can be used as presented, and others contain ideas which will have to be adapted and adjusted to fit specific populations. A very wide range of activities, ideas, suggestions, and experiences is presented here, and it is hoped that such a reference will be of use in a variety of settings serving the elderly.

BOOKS

Barnes, E.K. & Shore, H.H. *Holiday programming for long-term care facilities.* Denton, TX: Center for Studies in Aging, North Texas State University, 1977.

The author would like to thank activities personnel of nursing homes in the Seattle, Washington area for their suggestions and additions to this reference list, which appeared previously in *Activities, Adaptation & Aging* 7(2). It is reprinted here to complement this special issue.

Bennett, R. *Aging, isolation, and resocialization.* New York: Van Nostrand, 1980.

Bertolin, B.H. *Tidbits of useful information in rehabilitation nursing.* Rehabilitation Nursing Programs, Good Samaritan Hospital, 407 14th Ave. SE, Puyallup, WA 98371.

Bogen, M. *Leisure programming for older adults: An activities guide.* Denton, TX: Center for Studies in Aging, North Texas State University, 1981.

Brennan, J. *Memories, dreams, and thoughts: A guide to mental stimulation.* American Health Care Association, 1981.

Burnside, I.M. *Working with the elderly: Group processes and techniques* (2nd Ed.). Monterey, CA: Wadsworth Health Sciences Press, 1984.

Burnside, I.M. *Nursing and the aged.* New York: McGraw-Hill, 1981.

Caplow-Lindner, E., Harpaz, L., & Samberg, S. *Therapeutic dance and movement: Expressive activities for older adults.* New York: Human Sciences Press, 1979.

Case, M. *Recreation for blind adults.* Springfield, Ill: C.C. Thomas, 1966.

Chapman, F.M. *Recreational activities for the handicapped.* New York: Ronald Press, 1960.

Corbin, H.D. *Recreation leadership.* Englewood Cliffs, NJ: Prentice-Hall, 1959.

Danford, H.G. *Creative leadership in recreation.* Boston: Allyn & Bacon, 1970.

Duran, D.B. & Duran, C.A. *The new encyclopedia of successful program ideas.* New York: Association Press (YMCA), 1967.

Eisenberg, H. & Eisenberg, L. *How to help folks have fun.* New York: Association Press (YMCA), 1954.

Falkener, E. *Games ancient and oriental and how to play them.* New York: Dover Publications, 1961.

Fish, H.H. *Activities programs for senior citizens.* New York: Parker Pub., 1971.

Frankel, L.J. & Richard, B.B. *Be alive as long as you live.* Charleston, W.Va.: Preventicare Publications, 1977.

Gould, E. & Gould, L. *Crafts for the elderly.* Springfield, Ill: C.C. Thomas, 1971.

Gunn, S.L. & Peterson, C.A. *Therapeutic recreation program design.* Englewood Cliffs, NJ: Prentice-Hall, 1978.

Hamill, C.M. & Oliver, M.A. *Therapeutic activities for the handicapped elderly*. London: Aspen, 1980.

Harbert, A.S. & Ginsberg, L.H. *Human services for older adults: Concepts and skills*. Belmont, CA: Wadsworth, 1979.

Harbin, E.O. *The fun encyclopedia*. New York: Abingdon Press, 1940.

Hardy, R.E. & Cull, J.G. *Organization and administration of service programs for the older American*. Springfield, Ill: C.C. Thomas, 1975.

Hastings, L. *Complete handbook of activities and recreational programs for nursing homes*. Englewood Cliffs, NJ: Prentice-Hall, 1981.

Hawley, E.M. *Recreation is fun: A handbook on hospital recreation and entertainment*. New York: American Theatre Wing Inc., 1949.

Holdeman, E. *A guide for the activity coordinator in a skilled nursing facility*. Sacramento, CA: State Department of Health, 1975.

Hooker, S. *Caring for elderly people: Understanding and practical help*. London: Routledge & Kegan Paul, 1976.

Hunt, V.V. *Recreation for the handicapped*. Englewood Cliffs, NJ: Prentice-Hall, 1955.

Jacobs, B. (Ed.). *Working with the at-risk older person: A resource manual*. Washington, DC: National Council on the Aging, 1981.

Judd, M.W. *Why bother, he's old and confused*. Winnipeg, Manitoba: Winnipeg Municipal Hospital, 1974.

Kay, J.G. *Crafts for the very disabled and handicapped for all ages*. Springfield, Ill: C.C. Thomas, 1977.

Keddie, K.M.G. *Action with the elderly: A handbook for relatives and friends*. Oxford: Pergamon Press, 1978.

Kleemeier, R.W. *Aging and leisure*. New York: Oxford University Press, 1961.

Kubie, S.H. *Group work with the aged*. New York: International Universities Press, 1953.

Kurtz, R.H. *Manual for homes for the aged*. Recreation Service. Federation of Protestant Welfare Agencies, New York, 1965.

Laker, M. *Nursing home activities for the handicapped*. Springfield, Ill: C.C. Thomas, 1980.

Lonergan, E.C. *Group intervention: How to begin and maintain groups in medical and psychiatric settings.* New York: Jason Aronson, 1982.

Lucas, C. *Recreational activity development for the aging in homes, hospitals, and nursing homes.* Springfield, Ill: C.C. Thomas, 1962.

Macheath, J.A. *Activity, health, and fitness in old age.* New York: St. Martin's Press, 1984.

McDonald, W. *An old guy who feels good.* Ol'McDonald Press, PO Box 422, Berkeley, CA 94701, 1978.

Merrill, T. *Activities for the aged and infirm.* Springfield, Ill: C.C. Thomas, 1967.

Merrill, T. *Party packets for hospitals and homes.* Springfield, Ill: C.C. Thomas, 1970.

Merrill, T. *Discussion topics for oldsters in nursing homes.* Springfield, Ill: C.C. Thomas, 1974.

Perry, C.A. *Community center activities.* New York: Russell Sage Foundation, 1916.

Rosenberg, M. *Sixty-plus and fit again: Exercises for older men and women.* New York: M. Evans & Co., 1977.

Schuckman, T. *Aging is not for sissies.* Philadelphia: Westminster Press, 1975.

Shivers, J.S. & Fait, H.F. *Recreational service for the aging.* Philadelphia: Lea & Febiger, 1980.

Vannier, M. *Methods and materials in recreational leadership.* Philadelphia: W.B. Saunders, 1956.

Vickery, F.E. *Creative programming for older adults: A leadership training guide.* New York: Association Press (YMCA), 1972.

Vickery, F.E. *Old and growing.* Springfield, Ill: C.C. Thomas, 1978.

Wehman, P. & Schleier, S. *Leisure programming for handicapped persons.* Baltimore: University Park Press, 1981.

Weiner, M.B., Brok, A.J. & Snadowsky, A.M. *Working with the aged.* Englewood Cliffs, NJ: Prentice-Hall, 1978.

Wetzler, M.A. & Feil, N. *Validation therapy with disoriented aged who use fantasy.* E. Feil Productions, 4614 Prospect Ave., Cleveland, OH 44103, 1977.

Williams, A. *Recreation for the aging.* New York: Association Press (YMCA), 1953.

Witt, J., Campbell, M., & Witt, P. *Therapeutic group activities for leisure education.* Washington, DC: Hawkins and Associates, 1979.

————. *Pets in the nursing home.* Olympia, WA: Bureau of Nursing Home Affairs, Department of Social and Health Services, 1983.

————. *Resources for the aging: An action handbook* (2nd Ed.). New York: Community Action Program of the National Council on Aging, 1969.

————. *Recreation activities for adults.* New York: Association Press (YMCA), 1950.

PUBLICATIONS OF POTENTIALS DEVELOPMENT FOR HEALTH AND AGING SERVICES, INC.
(BUFFALO, NY)

Cornish, P. *Activities for the frail aged.*

Dickey, H. *Care center college.*

Dickey, H. *Activities from A to Z.*

Dickey, H. *Feelings.*

Dickey, H. *Reality and the senses.*

Dickey, H. *Swinging seniors.*

Feil, N. *Validation/fantasy therapy.*

Fiedler, A. *Memory sharing: Group programs for older adults.*

Frank, A. *Had stroke—still kicking.*

Garbach, L. & Pardo, A. *Exercises can be fun.*

Gordon, L., DePeters, J., & Wertman, A. *The magic of music.*

Griffin, P. *Guide to cooking projects in retirement and convalescent homes: Pat's practical palate program.*

Harmon, B. *How to get a drama off the ground and out on the town.*

Nelson, P.A. *The first year: A retirement journal.*

Quigley, P. *Creative writing I: A handbook for teaching wherever older adults gather.*

Quigley, P. *Those were the days* (life review).

Sullivan, M. *Where does your garden grow?*

Thornton, S. & Fraser, V. *Understanding "senility": A lay person's guide.*

Vieillard, M. *It is not as late as you think.*
Wade, S.C. *Mini-maxi parties.*

PUBLICATIONS OF THE HAWORTH PRESS
(NEW YORK)

Cusack, O. & Smith, E. *Pets and the elderly: The therapeutic bond.* 1984.

Foster, P. (Ed.). *Activities & the "well elderly".* 1983.

Kaminsky, E. (Ed.). *The use of reminiscence: New ways of working with older adults.* 1984.

Saul, S. (Ed.). *Groupwork with the frail elderly.* 1983.

Thurman, A. & Piggins, C.A. *Drama activities with older adults: A handbook for leaders.* 1982.

Weiss, J.C. *Expressive therapy with elders and the disabled: Touching the heart of life.* 1984.

Williams, J. & Downs, J.C. *Educational activity programs for older adults.* 1984.

JOURNAL ARTICLES

Blayney, J. Recreation—That important but often forgotten treatment in the total care of the long-term resident. *Alabama Journal of Medical Sciences,* 1975, 12, 210–212.

Burnside, I.M. Long-term group work with the hospitalized aged. *Gerontologist,* 1971, 11, 213–218.

Comstock, R.L., Mayers, R.L., & Folsom, J.C. Simple physical activities for the elderly. *Hospital & Community Psychiatry,* 1969, 20, 377–380.

Cozart, E.S. & Evashwick, C. Developing a recreational program for patients in a rural nursing home. *Public Health Reports,* 1978, 98, 369–374.

Curley, J.S. An activities program in a long term care facility. *Quality Review Bulletin,* 1981, 7, 12–18.

Kartman, L.L. Therapeutic group activities in nursing homes. *Health and Social Work,* 1979, 4, 135–144.

McClanahan, L.E. Recreational programs for nursing home residents: The importance of patient characteristics and environmental arrangements. *Therapeutic Recreation Journal,* 1973, 7, 26–31.

McClanahan, L.E. & Risley, T.R. Design of living environments for nursing home residents: Increasing participation in recreation activities. *Journal of Applied Behavioral Analysis,* 1975, 8, 261–268.

McClanahan, L.E. & Risley, T.R. A store for nursing home residents. *Nursing Homes,* 1973, 22, 10/11–29.

McClanahan, L.E. & Risley, T.R. Activities and materials for severely disabled geriatric patients. *Nursing Homes,* 1975, 24, 10–13.

McClanahan, L.E. & Risley, T.R. Design of living environments for nursing home residents: Recruiting attendance at activities. *Gerontologist,* 1974, 14, 236–240.

McCormack, D. & Whitehead, A. The effect of providing recreational activities on the engagement level of long-stay geriatric patients. *Age and Aging,* 1981, 10, 287–291.

Morgan, D.M. Community outreach in long-term care. *Dimensions of Health Services,* 1982, 59, 21–22.

Novick, L.J. Senile patients need diverse programming. *Dimensions of Health Services.* 1982, 59, 25–26.

Powell, L., Felce, D., Jenkins, & Lunt, B. Increasing engagement in activity of residents in old peoples' homes by providing an indoor gardening activity. *Behavioral Research and Therapy,* 1979, 17, 127–135.

Quiltch, H.R. Purposeful activity increase in a ward through programmed recreation. *Journal of the American Geriatrics Society,* 1974, 22, 226–229.

Rapelje, J.C. & Ventresca, D. Intergenerational programs—Untapped ideas. *Dimensions in Health Services,* 1982, 59, 28–29.

Rogers, J.C., Weinstein, J.M., & Figone, J.J. The interest checklist: An empirical assessment. *American Journal of Occupational Therapy,* 1978, 32, 628–630.

Stabler, N. The use of groups in day care centers for older adults. *Social Work with Groups,* 1981, 4, 49–58.

JOURNALS

Activity Director's Guide (monthly newsletter), c/o Eymann Publications Inc., PO Box 3577, Reno, NV 89505.

The Good Old Days, PO Box 428, Seabrook, NH 03874.

Parks and Recreation Resources, National Park and Recreation Association.

Therapeutic Recreation Journal, National Therapeutic Recreation Association.

Things to Do Monthly (monthly newsletter), c/o J. Lipman, PO Box 28132, Atlanta, GA 30358.

Effects of Institutionalization Upon Residents of Extended Care Facilities

Judith E. Voelkl

ABSTRACT. Many activity personnel talk about the difficulties of motivating residents to independently choose and participate in scheduled activities. The results of the research on learned helplessness and instrumental passivity provide activity personnel with a number of suggestions on how to decrease residents' dependent behaviors. As activity personnel structure the environment so residents perceive control, they may start to observe residents taking a more active role in activity groups and independently engaging in unscheduled leisure pursuits.

Helping professionals working in extended care facilities are continually challenged to enhance the quality of residents' lives. When discussing the challenge of their work, activity personnel frequently mention the difficulties of motivating residents to independently choose and participate in scheduled activities. Many activity staff discuss the frustration of residents never independently engaging in unscheduled leisure pursuits. Considering that many staff voice difficulties in motivating residents, one begins to wonder what causes residents to display passive and/or dependent behaviors. Is it possible that the environment affects the behavior of residents? In what ways does the helping professional affect residents' behavior? These unanswered questions concerning residents' passive behaviors prompted an investigation into the effects of institutionalization.

The author wishes to acknowledge and thank David R. Austin, Associate Professor, Indiana University, and Pauline N. Voelkl for their assistance in the preparation of this manuscript.

While reviewing literature pertaining to the negative effects of institutionalization, the theory of learned helplessness and the instrumental passivity hypothesis were continually noted. Both theories attempt to examine and explain the effects of loss of control for residents of extended care facilities. Perhaps, through examining these theories, we can begin to modify the negative effects of institutionalization. In order to clearly understand each theory, they will be separately presented along with corresponding research. The last section of this paper will discuss the implications of the theories for activity staff in extended care facilities.

LEARNED HELPLESSNESS

Learned helplessness theory was originally derived from learning theories and those of B. F. Skinner (Seligman, 1975). The theory is based on the belief that through uncontrollable outcomes and experiences people learn to believe they do not have control over the outcome of their behavior (Abramson, Garber, Seligman, 1980). Individuals experiencing learned helplessness may display emotional, cognitive, and motivational deficits (Seligman, 1975). An example would be when a nursing home resident initially takes an active role in resident council meetings. The resident council may be concerned with scheduling trips into the community and this particular resident may have a variety of suggestions. If several months pass and no scheduled out trips take place, the resident may begin to have difficulty thinking of any solutions to problems and may take a less active role in the resident council meetings. The resident begins to learn that his or her behavior does not affect the outcome. As a final outcome of learned helplessness, the resident might show signs of deprssion, perhaps isolation and/or lack of interest in any activities in the facility.

The learned helplessness theory draws from attribution theory in order to best explain the generality, chronicity, and type of helplessness symptoms (Abramson, Garber, Seligman, 1980). When utilizing attribution theory and learned helplessness, we need to consider if the individual attributes the uncontrollability of situations to internal (personal abilities) or external factors (environmental conditions). Additionally, one needs to consider if the condition is occurring in a stable or unstable environment. A stable environment is seen as one in which uncontrollable outcomes will not change, whereas an unstable environment is one in which the outcome will change in time. A nursing home is usually seen as a stable environment, for daily activities are very regimented and most residents do not anticipate leaving the facility. The chronicity of learned helplessness is also dependent upon whether the individual views the uncontrollability as only occurring during a specific event or views uncontrolled outcomes as being very global and affecting many aspects of his or her life. Individuals who attribute uncontrollability to internal, stable and global factors experience a more chronic and intense learned helplessness than those individuals who attribute uncontrollability to external, unstable and specific factors (Abramson, Garber, Seligman, 1980).

For instance, consider a resident council meeting where a resident was unable to get the leader or any other resident to listen to suggestions for a special event. The resident experiencing chronic, intense learned helplessness may believe that he or she lacked the ability to express or present ideas in any type of setting. Whereas the resident experiencing learned helplessness that was situation specific and externally based, may have thought the meeting was difficult for the leaders and disorganized. As can be seen from these examples, previous experiences and the general outlook one has about the world affects the intensity and chronicity of the learned helplessness a person experiences.

RESEARCH ON PERCEIVED CONTROL

A number of research projects investigating the effects of perceived control have been completed with nursing home residents. Most of the research mentions Seligman's learned helplessness theory as a reason for investigating the effects of control (Langer and Rodin, 1976; Schultz, 1976). Overall, the research does show that individuals who perceive that they have control in their environment show higher levels of physical ability, mental alertness, and general level of life satisfaction than individuals who do not perceive control. Possibly, through perceived control, learned helplessness can be prevented, or a degree of reversal in the helplessness process might occur.

Several studies have been completed in which nursing home residents are provided with opportunities to independently care for an object such as a bird feeder or plant (Langer and Rodin, 1976; Banziger and Roush, 1983). The bird feeder and plant were used as a means to provide the residents with perceived control. The experimental group and the control group (which was not provided with an opportunity to care for a plant or bird feeder) were rated in terms of physical ability, socialization and life satisfaction. Both studies showed that the group provided with an opportunity to experience control displayed higher levels of interpersonal activity, physical activity, and life satisfaction. Rodin and Langer (1977) completed a follow-up study which found that over an 18 month period the group provided with responsibility displayed higher health and activity patterns and their mortality rate was lower than the non-treatment group.

Another study showed that residents of nursing homes appear not to need to continually exercise their control in order to favorably respond to perceived control. Rodin (1980) went into a nursing home to investigate how perceived control would reduce the existing tension between staff and residents. The nursing staff expressed irritation and anger over residents continually calling for assistance. Rodin (1980) arranged for each resident to have an alarm clock and assigned a daily 15 minute period in which they could continually call the nursing staff for any reason. Initially, residents exercised their control by calling nursing staff to their rooms for reasons considered trivial. As time passed, residents called staff only for important reasons. The results suggest that control does not have to be continually exercised to produce benefits but benefits result from the simple knowledge that one has control.

Whether an individual attributes behavior to internal or external factors has been shown to have a significant effect on socialization and physical ability (Rodin, 1980). Nursing home residents who were given environmental (external) explanations for the source of their problems showed an increase in active participation and sociability over residents who were given no explanation or given information to argue against physical decline in aging. Environmental explanations decrease the likelihood that residents attribute their behaviors to aging. An example of an environmental explanation would be if a resident felt tired, the fatigue was stated to result from awakening at 5:30 a.m., not due to old age (Rodin, 1980). Environmental explanations for physical changes might prevent residents from labeling themselves as old and might prevent the breakdown of residents' self concept. When residents attribute physical deficits to external factors, their decline is not seen as a personal deficit. Therefore, individuals attributing physical deficits to external factors are less likely to develop feelings of personal helplessness.

The studies cited highlight the need for nursing home employees to consider ways to provide residents with perceived control. Overall, perceived control is shown to play an important role in residents' life satisfaction.

INSTRUMENTAL PASSIVITY

The instrumental passivity hypothesis is based on the operant learning models (Baltes, Skinner, 1983). The operant learning model is based on the belief that individuals repeat behaviors for which they are rewarded and decrease behaviors for which they are not rewarded. Baltes and Skinner (1983) found that residents of extended care facilities are offered rewards for certain types of behavior. "Independent, active, obviously control-taking behaviors are discouraged, ignored, or punished, whereas passive dependent behaviors are attended to, reinforced and encouraged." (Baltes, Skinner, 1983, p. 1014–1015). Instrumental passivity hypothesis views dependent behaviors of nursing home residents as resulting from environmental support (Baltes, Honn, Barton, Orzech, Lago, 1983). Possibly, the individual experiencing instrumental passivity may be responding to experience control within the environment. Passive, dependent behaviors may be displayed in order to elicit feedback from staff in extended care facilities.

OPERANT OBSERVATIONAL RESEARCH

Operant observational research in extended care facilities studies the naturally occurring behavior sequences between residents, staff and visitors. A majority of the research utilizing an operant observational design is implemented in order to provide a foundation to understand the dynamics of interactions in extended care facilities and to ultimately allow for the design of optional environments (Baltes and Barton, 1977). Observational research on the social environment of extended care facilities has been completed in order to provide more information on the instrumental passivity hypothesis (Baltes, Honn, Barton, Orzech, Lago, 1983).

Baltes, Honn, Barton, Orzech and Lago (1983) studied the behavior of forty residents in a nursing home. Trained observers recorded residents' behavior and the response of social partners. Generally, it was found that residents who displayed independent personal maintenance received no reactions from the social ecology. Residents constructively engaged received intermittent support. Residents engaged in dependent maintenance behavior received the greatest amount of support from social partners. Barton, Baltes and Orzech (1980) found similar results when examining staff and resident interactions during morning care.

Many professionals who work in institutional settings would not be surprised at the results of studies utilizing operant observational techniques. The institutional setting is one which attempts to set a routine and establish expectation for appropriate behavior in order to have a smooth running operation. Furthermore, the results of the studies mentioned may be partially due to staffing patterns in extended care facilties. If a facility operates with a small staff, they may only have time to interact with residents who display dependent behaviors due to functional decrements. Another consideration is liability. Staff might encourage dependent behaviors due to concerns over possible accidents when residents are attempting a task independently. This is of particular concern if residents display poor judgment concerning their abilities. These possible explanations for staff supporting dependent behaviors are not an attempt to condone such interaction.

Rather, through explanations and results of research, we can begin to understand where and why changes must be made in extended care facilities.

IMPLICATIONS FOR ACTIVITY STAFF

Learned helplessness and instrumental passivity are closely related. The end point of each theory occurs in the same place—perceptions of loss of control and passivity. Each theory focuses on the individual's experience in the social environment. The difference between the theories occurs in the way the individual learns to display dependent or passive behavior. Learned helplessness is a product of noncontingency or experiencing no personal control over outcomes and events (Abramson, Garber, Seligman, 1980). Whereas instrumental passivity views dependent behaviors of residents resulting from the support of staff and significant others (Baltes, Honn, Barton, Orzech, Lago, 1983). Regardless of the differences between the two theories, we can utilize both theories to better understand residents' behavior.

Activities are a natural arena in which independent behaviors are stressed and can be used to combat the negative effects of learned helplessness and instrumental passivity. Since activity departments focus on wellness and assisting clients to achieve maximum potential, the activities provided naturally lend themselves to reinforce independent behaviors of clients. Activities can provide positive experiences, role continuity, and reinforcement of the whole person rather than the dependent individual.

In order to fully understand the impact the environment has on a resident, it is necessary to understand how the individual views himself or herself in relation to the world. Staff can begin to understand a resident's behavior by talking to the resident and to the family members. Many of the ways in which a person reacts to the world are due to past experiences. Information on what a resident attributes his or her behavior to, how the individual reacts to loss, and what roles have been and are currently important can be useful when attempting to understand a resident's behavior. When staff have a clear understanding of a resident's behavior and perceptions, they can then choose the most effective means of interaction and can also set realistic goals for future behavior.

The initial process of institutionalization can result in an individual experiencing learned helplessness. Staff need to provide opportunities for residents to make choices and experience control beginning at the time of admission. When possible, it is important to involve residents in the development of their treatment plan. The treatment plan provides residents with the knowledge of areas in which they can realistically improve. Involvement in the treatment planning phase also allows residents to be treated as functioning adults responsible for their care rather than being cared for by staff. Lastly, involving residents in the treatment planning encourages all staff to treat residents as individuals. Treating each person as an individual and reinforcing their strengths can be a powerful means of decreasing learned helplessness and instrumental passivity.

When attempting to decrease dependent behaviors, it is necessary to sequence activities so that participants are able to have successful experiences. It is extremely important to make sure an activity is structured to meet the functional level of the residents. If an activity is too difficult, the residents may feel a lack of effectiveness or control. On the other hand, if an activity is routine or non-challenging, the resident will lose interest. As residents' functional level changes, the level of activity in which they participate must also change. Hopefully, as residents are appropriately challenged and experience success, they can begin to view themselves as effective individuals. Successful experience also provides a perfect opportunity for staff to reinforce active behaviors. Through positive reinforcement and successful experiences, residents may begin to independently engage in activities.

In conclusion, the theory of learned helplessness and the instrumental passivity hypothesis are two possible explanations for residents' passive and dependent behaviors. The results of the research on learned helplessness and instrumental passivity provide activity personnel with a number of suggestions on how to decrease residents' dependent behaviors. Activity personnel can provide successful experiences, positive feedback, and involve residents in the treatment planning process in order to provide residents an environment in which they perceive control. As residents begin to feel more effective and perceive control in their environment, they may start to take a more active role in activity groups and independently engage in unscheduled leisure pursuits.

REFERENCES

Abramson, L. Y., Garber, J., Seligman, M. E. (1980). Learned Helplessness in Humans: An Attributional Analysis. In Garber, J. and Seligman, M. E. (Eds.), *Human Helplessness: Theory and Applications* (pp. 3–34). New York: Academic Press.

Baltes, M. M. (1982). Environmental Factors in Dependency Among Nursing Home Residents: A Social Ecology Analysis. In T. A. Wills (Ed.), *Basic Processes in Helping Relationships* (pp. 405–425). New York: Academic Press.

Baltes, M. M., Honn, S., Barton, E. M., Orzech, M. J., Lago, D. (1983). On the Social Ecology of Dependence and Independence in Elderly Nursing Home Residents: A Replication and Extension. *Journal of Gerontology, 38* (5), 556–564.

Baltes, M. M., Skinner, E. A. (1983). Cognitive Performance Deficits and Hospitalization: Learned Helplessness, Instrumental Passivity, or What? *Journal of Personality and Social Psychology, 45* (5), 1013–1016.

Banziger, G., Roush, S. (1983). Nursing Homes for the Birds: A Control-Relevant Intervention with Bird Feeders. *The Gerontologist, 23* (5), 527–531

Barton, E. M., Baltes, M. M., Orzech, M. J. (1980). Etiology of Dependence in Older Nursing Home Residents During Morning Care: The Role of Staff Behavior. *Journal of Personality and Social Psychology, 38* (3), 423–431.

Langer, E. J., Rodin, J. (1976). The Effects of Choice and Enhanced Personal Responsibility for the Aged: A Field Experiment in An Institutional Setting. *Journal of Personality and Social Psychology, 34* (2), 191–198.

Rodin, J. (1980). Managing the Stress of Aging: The Role of Control and Coping. In Leving, S. (Ed.), *Coping and Health* (pp. 171–202).

Rodin, J., Langer, E. J. (1977). Long-Term Effects of a Control-Relevant Intervention With the Institutionalized Aged. *Journal of Personality and Social Psychology, 35* (12), 897–902.

Schultz, R. (1976). Effects of Control and Predictability on the Physical and Psychological Well-Being of the Institutionalized Aged. *Journal of Personality and Social Psychology, 33* (5), 563–573.

Seligman, Martin E. (1975). *Helplessness: On Depression, Development, and Death.* San Francisco: W. H. Freeman and Company.

A Protocol for Recreation and Socialization Programs for the Aged

Michael J. Salamon

ABSTRACT. This paper explores some of the components and parameters necessary for the successful achievement of the goal for recreation and socialization programs. This goal, helping older adults maintain the highest possible level of physical and mental functioning, is facilitated when group leaders provide a variety of programs and encourage participation. Participation is, in turn, enhanced by using a variety of motivational techniques. Success is measured not in terms of simple attendance, but by the ability of a group to achieve its stated goals.

Programs for recreation and socialization serve a therapeutically beneficial role for the aged (McCormack & Whithead, 1983). These programs help to reduce stress and the sense of helplessness and hopelessness so often found among the aged. They also help to improve an individual's self-concept, enhance one's sense of self-worth and raise the individual's level of life satisfaction (Hastings, 1981; Macheath, 1984).

This paper establishes some basic parameters for providing recreation and socialization programs for older adults. The importance of programs and their conceptualization according to categories is presented. These are then followed by special motivational techniques and additional considerations in making the program a success. Often, because of this concern for

Michael J. Salamon, PhD is Director, Adult Development Center: a Health Care & Geriatric consulting firm. Please address inquiries to: 920 Broadway, Suite 1-A, Woodmere, New York 11598.

The author wishes to thank the anonymous reviewers for their constructive criticisms.

the success of a specific program, activities specialists lose sight of the greater goal of programming.

Staff members who provide programs of recreation and socialization to the aged have one major goal, and that is to help the participants remain as physically and mentally active and alert as possible. This one goal, however, is quite broad and consists of many components. One component is the staff's professional involvement in planning and programming. Staff members who provide recreation and socialization need to project a sense of enthusiasm, approach programming with ingenuity and have a particularly warm feeling toward the program participants.

The staff must also be able to provide a wide range of programs while at the same time remaining responsive to the needs of each individual (Salamon, in press). Another component of the goal of maintaining well-being through recreation is the structuring of program activities to reflect the varied interests of the participants. To accomplish this a set of parameters must be established which provides structure for the programming. Without structure it would be impossible to know if the participants interests and needs are being met. The first step in establishing parameters may be to specify criteria for evaluation.

One particularly easy evaluative method is the number of individuals in attendance at a particular activity or program. The success of a recreational or socialization activity can not, however, always be measured by the number of people who attend. If groups are small or attendance static, success can be measured subjectively by the feelings generated in the participants within a specific activity group. Often these feelings expressed to group leaders or administrators are described as a sense of cohesiveness or belonging (Burnside, 1984). When this feeling is reported as existing within a group the evaluation is a positive one.

Another measure of success is whether or not, having achieved the feelings of cohesiveness, the group can move on toward achieving its own objectives. These objectives are easily stated and take the form of: can the dance group learn a new dance, can the social action group arrange to have a politician come and speak, and so forth.

The second parameter of helping participants remain mentally and physically active is related to the types of activities which are offered as well as the socialization which goes along with a particular activity. Individuals should be exposed to varied activities as well as individuals who attend these activities. Not only does this method of cross-programming increase the likelihood of expanding an individual's interest, but it exposes him/her to other persons, thereby increasing the likelihood of expanding his/her social network. If a large party is being organized the arts and crafts group can prepare the decorations, the social action group can handle the invitations, while the drama group can prepare a short show for the affair. All of the groups have their own goals, but all must work together and can share the benefits of the experience.

To better understand the parameters of programming it is necessary to discuss activities according to categories such that planning can be arranged across them. Szekais (this issue) suggests that there are six different categories of activities. For the present purposes, however, it is appropriate to divide general activities programming into four categories (Salamon & Nichol, 1983). The four categories are:

A. physical activities, which include exercise and dancing groups as well as sports and similar physically intensive pastimes;
B. socialization groups, where mental or emotional involvement is necessary, including resident council meetings, sing-alongs, current events, literature and choral groups;
C. board games, which are not physically or mentally demanding, such as bingo or simple crafts projects; and,
D. a general category of special activities, such as parties and other similar special events.

PHYSICAL ACTIVITIES

In each of the four activity categories, techniques for enhancement of individual's participation within the group may be specified. In the category of physical activities, group leaders have the responsibility of showing program participants how to "get in touch" with their bodies. A feeling of control must be re-established for the elderly. They are often weak and lethargic and possibly even lazy. Physical activity groups can help to sharpen not only one's body, but one's mind as well. The group leader can communicate this to group participants by feeling at ease and encouraging participants to feel the same.

This technique of encouraging participants extends to those who have limited physical abilities. Not only is limited activity better than a sedentary life style for physical reasons, but the encouragement given often enhances the participants' self-esteem to the point where they can begin to take a more positive and healthy view of themselves. ·

One common form of physical activity is exercise. Exercise programs generally consist of three parts, the warm-up, period of peak work and the cooling off time. The warm-up period is a time where the participants stretch and loosen up. During the period of peak work the most strenuous exercises are performed. The cooling off period should be a time devoted not simply to relaxing, but should also be a time when the group leader talks about the benefits of exercise and a healthy body.

Dance is a physical activity that often has a broad appeal. Dances and dancing are generally associated with joyous occasions. Dancing also encourages direct socialization with other people (Caplow-Linder et al., 1979). Dance instructors should not forget or minimize these points by looking at the dance group as simply another activity. Group leaders should wear brightly colored clothing, set a party atmosphere and dance with as many participants as possible. The first dance should be an easy one but at an upbeat tempo. Like exercise, the first few dances can be considered a period of warm up. The peak period in exercise does not mean that only fast dances are played, rather that new steps are taught. During the cooling off period slow dances are once again played and the group leader discusses the types of music and dance steps to be performed at the next group meeting.

Physical activities within an overall program encourage and enhance socialization by providing a forum for interaction with older participants. A physical activity which promotes a sense of continuity with the social sphere outside of the activities program is the outing or trip. Participants are afforded the opportunity to interact with individuals in settings they are not often exposed to. Some guidelines for these trips include knowing total walking distance involved and distance to toilet facilities, preparing box lunches and snacks, knowing if show seats are close enough for the actors to be seen and heard and other similar considerations necessary for the comfort of the particular group.

SOCIALIZATION GROUPS

Socialization groups stimulate mental awareness and encourage social interaction through discourse helping individuals achieve a sense of accomplishment (Stabler, 1981). These groups are also particularly useful in alleviating the sense of loneliness often found among the aged (Burnside, 1984). Socialization groups can focus on a variety of discussion topics such as retirement problems, life experiences, current events and even socio-therapy such as problem solving or supportive counseling.

Regardless of the topic of the group, several basic techniques may be employed. Preparing for a socialization group requires advertising the program several weeks before its initial inception. This may be done via the local media as well as posters and invitations (Salamon & Charytan, 1984).

Socialization groups are often best conducted in a round table format. This format heightens the sense of participation among the group members. Rules for participation in these groups should be made clear. Perhaps the most important rule is to allow only one person at a time to speak. The group leader may find it necessary to direct the conversation toward individuals who tend not to participate often enough and away from individuals who are too controlling. This should be done in a gentle but firm fashion. Socialization group leaders must always be prepared in advance for the topic under discussion. While it may be difficult to prepare for a group discussing emotional loss, the leader should minimally have knowledge of referral sources if participants require more intensive emotional or psychological support.

A particularly useful group in the category of socialization groups is the political action committee. A political action committee encourages participants to continue to exercise their responsibilities as citizens. The committee can form smaller social action groups to deal with specific issues, arrange guest speakers or conduct straw poles.

Religious activities, including religious services, bible study and spiritual therapy, should all be provided for those who wish these activities. Programming for these activities can often be arranged through creative use of contact with religious institutions. Participants may be provided transportation to houses of worship or clerics may volunteer to attend specific activities at the program site.

Several music programs can be considered in the category of socialization groups. These include sing-alongs, music clubs and choral groups. Group leaders should allow group participants to select the music they find most inspiring. These groups require a cohesiveness and sense of discipline not found in other types of activities. As a result, it is important to encourage a sense of group oneness by encouraging a broad enough selection of music to satisfy the taste of all the participants and providing the discipline and structure necessary for group unity.

Another means of enhancing self-expression is arts and crafts. Complex art and craft activities that require concentration are considered in the category of socialization groups because of the mental involvement of the participants. The rewards of participation include completion of the task, display of the completed item, and when appropriate, sale of the item. In providing these activities group leaders should have all the necessary materials in a well-lit, properly ventilated work area. Leaders should also be familiar with the progression of steps toward completion of the project, and keeping instructions clear. A great deal of encouragement particularly for difficult tasks should be provided.

Despite the individual nature of some of these activities socialization takes place. Interactions occur between participants, and between group leaders and participants. A sense of success as well as a sense of pride is shared when goals are achieved.

BOARD GAMES

Board games are often viewed as being of less importance than the other categories of recreational activities. While these simple activities are not physically or mentally demanding, they do meet a variety of needs of the elderly. Group participation, while not necessarily socially interactive, does allow the participants to feel active and involved in a group. The activity itself may not require great mental concentration, but does require the participant to remain alert and aware of the proceeding. Individuals who are shy or unsure of their abilities have no difficulty taking part in a bingo game. Group leaders clearly have the responsibility to encourage participation in these activities. Individuals who are satisfied with their own participation tend to view attendance at these activities as an important daily goal.

SPECIAL EVENTS

Special events are activities that focus on a specific theme. These activities are not held on a daily, or even a regular basis. Included in these activities are birthday parties, award dinner, fashion shows and so forth. As mentioned above, group leaders should facilitate interaction between many groups when planning and conducting special events. Crafts groups can prepare the posters announcing the events as well as decorations and even the awards. The dance group, drama group and music group can all prepare entertainment. The interactions among usually disparate groups culminating in a highly successful special event is an extremely rewarding experience.

MOTIVATION

In the previous sections we have spoken of the responsibility of the group leader in several formats. There is one general overriding responsibility that a group activity leader has and that is to motivate the participants to attend the activities which are best suited for them. To do so requires a knowledge of the individual's skills, interests and physical abilities. Before the group leader can determine the individual's skills and level of abilities, the leader must develop rapport with the participants. This is done through positive verbal dialogue, knowing how the individuals like to be addressed and simply communicating with individuals on a one-to-one basis.

The interests of individuals can be ascertained by the use of interest inventories or questionnaires. This approach is very structured and direct. Another method is by starting a wide variety of programs at the facility encouraging individuals to attend, keeping records of attendance and noting who regularly attends which activities.

Frequent advertising, announcing and recognizing of participation are additional motivational techniques (Salamon, in press). Motivating individuals to participate often requires great creativity. Inviting guests or family members, or changing activity times may all be used to successfully motivate participation.

ADDITIONAL CONSIDERATIONS

There are several issues group leaders must be aware of in addition to the components mentioned above. To provide an appropriate program requires offering a wide variety of activities. As no single individual can be expected to be knowledgeable or conduct activities in all of the areas mentioned, a well-rounded staff must be available. The staff may consist of only one full-time individual responsible for all recreation and socialization programs. That individual's responsibility however should be supplemented by other part-time program specialists and volunteers.

The scheduling of activities is also an important consideration. No activity, unless it is a special activity or a long outing, should be scheduled for an entire morning or entire afternoon. Generally, activities last between 45 minutes and an hour and a half, occasionally up to two hours. The length, however, depends on the activity, the number of rest periods provided and the interest and stamina of the participants.

Group participants may usually be divided into two types. There are the core participants, active group members, and those who are often referred to as active observers or passive participants (Salamon, in press). The active participants are those who speak in the discussion groups or are the first to dance in the dance groups. Passive participants are individuals who sit away from the round table in the discussion group or watch the dancers in the dance group while they sit and just tap their feet. Both forms of participation, active and passive, are equally valid and group leaders should not minimize either form of participation. There are occasions when passive participants become active and active participants become passive. The need of the individual should always be respected in this regard.

The physical setting where activities are conducted is also a consideration for programming and planning. It is difficult to conduct a small discussion group in a large room where many people congregate and many other activities are being held. On the other hand, if no small quiet room is available, the manipulation of furniture to provide a secluded corner for the discussion may be an acceptable alternative. Simlarly, activities such as dancing, which attract a good number of individuals both as active and passive participants, cannot be held in small rooms. Group leaders must be aware of the programming needs and the availability of the physical plant to respond to these needs. Similarly, the tables, chairs, and lighting fixtures should all be designed to enhance the activity that is being conducted. Chairs should be sufficiently comfortable to allow participants to sit for the duration of the activity. The chairs should not be on wheels and should have arms so that group participants can easily lift themselves out of the chair at the end of the activity. Lighting should be bright but without glare. Florescent lights combined with natural sunlight often provide the best visual stimulation.

As stated previously, evaluation of the success of an activity is an important consideration. Three useful methods of evaluation are attendance records, group cohesiveness and the achievement of group goals. Of these methods, the best measure is the degree to which groups work together and are able to accomplish their stated goals.

SUMMARY

This paper described several components necessary for the establishment of a successful recreation and socialization program whose primary goal is to help participants remain physically and mentally active. Among these components are staff responsibility toward the group as well as the individual.

Group leaders should provide a broad range of activities including physical activities, socialization groups, board games and special events. They should also encourage participation using a variety of techniques. Some general techniques include establishing rapport, encouraging participation, advertising a program and knowing the needs, interests and abilities of individuals who attend. Group leaders are encouraged to be creative using part-time specialists and volunteers to enhance the ability to provide programs. They should not allow an activity to run for too long a period of time, respecting an individual's right to participate at their level of choice, and provide as comfortable a physical environment as possible.

REFERENCES

Burnside, I.M. (1984) *Working With the Elderly: Group Processes and Techniques,* *2nd Ed.* Monterey, California: Wadsworth Health Sciences Press.

Caplow-Lindner, E., Harpaz, L., & Samberg, S. (1979) *Therapeutic Dance and Movement: Expressive Activities for Older Adults.* New York: Human Sciences Press.

Hastings, L. (1981) *The Complete Handbook of Activities and Recreational Programs for Nursing Homes.* Englewood Cliffs, New Jersey: Prentice Hall.

Macheath, J.A. (1984) *Activity, Health, and Fitness in Old Age.* New York: St. Martins Press.

McCormack, D., & Whithead, A. (1981) The effect of providing recreational activities on the engagement level of long-stay geriatric patients. *Age and Aging, 10,* 287–291.

Salamon, M.J. (in press) *Basic Practices in Applied Gerontology.* New York: Springer Publishing Co.

Salamon, M.J., & Charytan, P. (1984) Sexuality workshops for the elderly. *Clinical Gerontologist, 2,* 25–34.

Salamon, M.J., & Nichol, A. (1982) Rx for recreation: Part of the doctor's role. *Aging, 333–334,* 18–22.

Stabler, N. (1981) The use of groups in day centers for older adults. *Social Work With Groups, 4,* 49–58.

Szekais, B. (this issue). Therapeutic individual activities with the impaired elderly. *Activities, Adaptation and Aging.*

A Humanistic Approach
to Old-Old People:
A General Model

Leonard Babins

ABSTRACT. The present article is designed to provide an overview of Validation Therapy. The purpose of this approach is to validate the uniqueness of Old-Old (80 years and older) disoriented residents, helping them regain their sense of dignity and self-worth without being judgmental. This approach was discussed in terms of two underlying principles. The first is that early emotional learning is retained in Old-Old persons despite cognitive deterioration. The second principle is based on Erik Erikson's Life Stages. It was suggested that Validation Therapy is a promising approach with disoriented elderly. Finally, further research in this area is needed and encouraged.

The following article is based on a conference given by Naomi Feil on Validation Therapy. Its objective is to provide an overview of this approach in order to encourage further investigations.

Feil's approach is similar to Carl Rogers' humanistic outlook in that it emphasizes the essential freedom and dignity of the individual. When the therapist is experiencing a positive acceptant attitude toward whatever the client is feeling or expressing at that moment, personal growth or change is more likely to occur. The helper encourages the helpee to express whatever immediate feeling is being experienced—

Leonard Babins, BA Honours Psychology is with McGill University, Montreal, Quebec.

The author wishes to thank Steven Merovitz for his recommendations in preparing this article. The ideas developed in this paper originated at a conference from Porcupine General Hospital, Timmons, Ontario, on Wednesday, December 5, 1984, given by Naomi Feil.

57

confusion, resentment, fear, anger, courage, or love (Rogers, 1977).

The purpose of the Feil method is to validate the uniqueness of elderly disoriented, institutionalized residents, helping them to regain their sense of dignity and self-worth focusing on unresolved feelings enabling them to work out life's unfinished conflicts. The meaning of validation is to acknowledge and respect the feelings of the person. In this approach the quality of the relationship between the helper and helpee is the actual therapy which is concerned with restoring the old aged person's self-esteem in their own terms without being judgmental.

There are two major principles underlying Validation Therapy. The first is that early emotional learning stays with a person in Old-Old age (80 years and older) despite the fact that cognitive learning deteriorates. An example of early emotional learning is when a 6-month old baby climbs on the stairs, prompting the mother to grab the child and angrily tell him not to climb.

More specifically, when the baby sees the mother, the optic nerve carries a "visual" message up to higher brain centers encoding a visual representation of the mother's anger. The auditory nerve carries the oral message associated with the mother's loud tone of voice. At the nerve endings synaptic changes occur when learning takes place. According to the contiguity theory, whenever a neuron A fires a neuron B, the A-B connection is strengthened. This message is carried to the muscles and glands in the body.

In the example cited above, the results are trembling of the limbs, sweating and increased heart rate. This occurs from the adrenal gland whose inner portion secretes a hormone on smooth muscles (Hebb, 1966). Ultimately, the outcome is that the child may cry, indicating that anxiety is present. Finally, the message goes from the muscles and glands back up to the higher brain centres and then learning is completed.

It is a circuit that is permanently embedded in the mind of the child who has learned that climbing or risk-taking, depending on how the situation is interpreted, will be punished by his mother. When this child grows up, although he may not have consciously retained his earlier learning, the memory can still be triggered by a similar event (Feil, 1984).

For example, this same person, now 90 years old with sensory deterioration, is suddenly forced to move to a new apartment which has very poor lighting. The early emotional memory of climbing the stairs is stimulated by the emotional similarity of the present situation. Intellectually, it has been forgotten, but emotionally and physiologically, the quick heart rate, sweating, the surge of ephinephrine from his adrenal glands, encourages him to respond in the present time as if it were the past.

The process of encoding precise sensory and emotional memories was discovered by Penefield (1950) who performed neurosurgery using an electrode placed on the temporal lobe of the brain. Patients experienced very vividly what happened when they were much younger. By stimulating different parts of the brain, he was able to map the brain artificially. By stimulating the temporal cortex, he established the link between present sensory perceptions and past experiences.

As aging occurs, there are many physiological changes that may result in an impairment in logical thinking. When this occurs, it has been suggested by Zaidel (1978) that non-rational or emotional outputs become heightened. For instance, during the dream state, one does not use logical thinking but non-rational eidetic images. These images help to restore events from the past.

Traditionally, according to D. O. Hebb (1966), both imagery and hallucination may be defined as the occurrence of perceptual processes in the absence of the stimulation which normally gives rise to the perception. We call it a "hallucination" when the subject perceives something that is not externally present. Allport (1928) suggested that the eidetic image is in the same class with memory image, it is recognized that eye movement has a positive, integrating role in memory images.

Similarly, Feil (1982) has termed the recreation of old memories as "seeing with the mind's eye." For example, if a 90 year old person never told her mother that she loved her, she may recreate her through eidetic imagery. This Old-Old person may have a feeling of guilt associated with these unresolved issues. In fact, Freud (1949), using the technique of classical psychoanalysis on younger patients, found that they projected into the therapeutic situation feelings and attitudes that occurred in their past. By recovering and recognizing these experiences and conflictual situations, modifications were possible.

Concerning Old-Old people, from our perspective, it is often concluded that they are demented when they reveal unresolved inner issues through eidetic imagery. The fact that certain feelings have been denied during adulthood may lead to a breakdown of defense mechanisms in old age. Often this denial or repression leads to a final retreat to fantasy and emotional behaviour when the individual is alone and dependent on others for activities of daily living. This stimulates the regression to childhood and unresolved feelings from this period (Verwoerdt, 1980). The concept of emotional expression forms the foundation of Validation Therapy.

One important factor that should be considered is the presence of regulators that enable Old-Old people to maintain their sense of orientation. During aging, brain cell atrophy occurs as well as a decrease in the amount of oxygen flowing to the brain. As a result of aging, there are neuroanatomical changes like neurofibrillary tangles throughout the neocortex and hippocampus that could affect behaviour (Reisberg, 1981).

Houts (1967) examined the results of autopsies on elderly people to determine the relationship between the patient's behaviour and the amount of brain damage. The findings were that many patients behave "normally" until the time of death, despite severe physiological damage. Others with relatively intact brain structures show marked disorientation (Aker, Walsh, Beam, 1977). Therefore, it is suggested here that the condition of the brain is not the only regulator of behaviour. Other regulators include psychological factors and coping mechanisms which determine how they relate to their environmental surroundings.

Feil (1984) has suggested that Old-Old disoriented cope in different ways. Some cope with their losses by freely associating different thoughts. Behaviourally, the Old-Old disoriented may produce illogical words and sentences, unusual sounds and meaningless hand and body movements (Peoples, 1982). This enables their attention to be taken away from the stress of their present reality. Usually their overt behaviour appears bizarre, and they are judged against the standards and values of a society which is no longer meaningful to them.

In fact, the Old-Old persons are coping in the most adaptive manner possible given their set of life experiences. Some patients withdraw, retreating to their own inner cosmos, or constantly dozing off in order to avoid reality, while others may resist or fight their helplessness by aggressive behaviour such as yelling, screaming and biting, resulting in their being tranquilized and restrained.

The second principle underlying Validation Therapy is based on Erik Erikson's Life Stages. During a person's lifetime, there are a number of stages, each of which offers a developmental crisis which an individual must face and which is crucial in determining their overall level of personality growth. Erikson (1963) defined the last stage of life as "ego integrity versus despair," and describes the possessor of integrity as being able to defend the dignity of his own lifestyle against different threats. The integrated person accepts his life's events and resolves his conflicts.

Feil (1982) and Peoples (1982) have pointed out that failure to resolve this stage means that the person will not be able to defend himself against both his physical and psychological losses. For instance, an 80 year old who, as a younger person, blamed other people for personal failures, may continue to blame people in the nursing home. This Old-Old person may think that the nurses are trying to poison her food, or that other residents are stealing her clothes. When this same individual was younger, her style of blaming others was never successfully resolved, although she was able to function well in society. Now that this person has reached Old-Old age, her losses create anxiety and she ultimately is left with a feeling of despair. Without the ability to resolve unfinished past conflicts, the individual vegetates until death (Feil, 1982).

Typically, rather than confirming the attitude of acceptance and worth, we apply labels that do not take into account a person's life experience. A climate of warmth and acceptance is not used to discover the person's perspective (Peoples, 1982).

Feil (1982) divided disorientation into four stages ranging from mild to severe disorientation. Each state is distinguishable on the basis of emotional characteristics, physical characteristics, and feelings that are experienced by people in that stage.

Validation Therapy has been found to be most successful with patients in stages two and three. (Interested readers should consult Feil (1982) for a more comprehensive discussion in this area.) Mental health professionals cannot change the reality about a person's life. Using Validation Therapy can help the Old-Old disoriented to grow in a genuine trusting relationship. Accepting the individual's right to be unique has been suggested by Watzlawick, Beavin & Jackson (1967), as probably the greatest single factor ensuring mental development and stability of persons in a relationship. Therefore, the primary goal of Validation Therapy is to give the person a sense of identity, dignity and self-worth by validating their feelings without analyzing and interpreting their actions.

In conclusion, an overview of the theory behind Validation Therapy has been presented, based on the work of N. Feil. The approach appears to be promising as an effective therapy in communicating and relating with Old-Old disoriented.

Finally, it should be stressed that research and increased attention is needed in this area in order to determine how the therapy can be more successfully implemented.

REFERENCES

Aker, J. B., Walsh, A. C., Beam, J. R. (1977). *Mental Capacity, Medical and Legal Aspects of the Aging.* New York: McGraw-Hill Book Co.

Allport, as cited in Nicholas, J. M. (1968). *Images, Perception and Knowledge,* (pp. 139–159). American Psychological Association.

Erikson, E. (1963). *Childhood and Society.* New York: W. W. Norton & Co.

Feil, N. W. From tapes based on conference from Porcupine General Hospital, Timmons, Ontario, December 5, 1984.

Feil, N. W. (1982). *V/F Validation The Feil Method: How to Help Disoriented Old-Old.* Cleveland: Edward Feil Productions.

Freud, S. (1949). *An Outline of Psychoanalysis.* New York: Norton.

Hebb, D. O. (1966). *A Textbook of Psychology.* Philadelphia: W. B. Saunders Company.

Houts, M. (1967). *Where Death Delights.* New York: Kurtis Brown.

Penefield, W. G. (1950). *The Cerebral Cortex of Man.* A Clinical Study of Localization of Function. New York: The MacMillan Company.

Peoples, M. (1982). *Validation Therapy Versus Reality Orientation as Treatment for Disoriented Institutionalized Elderly.* Unpublished Master's Thesis, College of Nursing, Akron, Ohio.

Reisberg, B. (1982). *A Guide to Alzheimer's Disease for Families, Spouses and Friends.* New York: The Free Press.

Rogers, C. (1977). *On Personal Power.* New York: Delacorte Press.

Verwoerdt, A. (1980). Anxiety, Dissociative and Personality Disorders in the Elderly. Chapter 16 in Busse, E. W., Blazer, D. G. *Handbook of Geriatric Psychiatry.* New York: Van Nostrand Reinhold Company.

Watzlawich, P., Beavin, J., Jackson, D. D. (1967). *Pragmatics of Human Communication.* New York: W. W. Norton & Co.

Zaidel, A. (1978). Concepts of Cerebral Dominance in the Split Brain in Busse, E. W. *Cerebral Correlates of Conscious Experience,* (pp. 263–284). Ellaster: North Holland.

"Worth Repeating"
Reality Orientation:
Full Circle

Geneva Scheihing Folsom

Reality orientation, a "psychological treatment approach in treating the problems of confused elderly people" and "the most widely researched of the psychological approaches to confusion,"[1] began in 1958 as a pilot rehabilitation program in one unit at Winter Veterans Administration Hospital, Topeka, Kansas. From a 24-year retrospective, we recognize that the strict medical model of geriatric care is only the core of effective programming for elderly and other clients with multiple problems who need long-term care or support.

Over time, reality orientation has been successfully employed as a vital part of changing long-term care custodial environments into more active treatment milieux, but packaging its broad and complex concepts for wide consumption has sometimes resulted in the addition of a clock, a calendar, an RO Board, and an RO Class which has been misinterpreted as an RO program.

The demographic imperatives and clinical realities of the aging veteran population in 1983 demand that we try to close the circle by reintegration of reality orientation as an essential part of individualized rehabilitation planning and tracking. Although reality orientation is specifically used to assist with problems of disorientation and confusion, "If I don't know

The author is Management Analyst, Quality Assurance Office, Veterans Administration Central Office, Washington, DC. Please address inquiries to: Quality Assurance Office (10QA1), V.A. Central Office, 810 Vermont Ave. N.W., Washington, DC.

This article is modified from a paper presented at a meeting of the Section on Geriatrics of the New York Academy of Medicine held December 14, 1983. This article originally appeared in *Bulletin of the New York Academy of Medicine*, Second Series, Vol. 61, No. 4, pp. 343–350, May 1985.

who I am, where I am, or what time of day or night it is, I am a nonperson."[2] The impact is global.

In 1951 I was one of the first music therapy interns at Winter Hospital; problems earlier identified today were the same, but the patient mix was reversed. We worked with acute psychiatric patients while the new field of psychiatry was rapidly developing under the auspices of the Menninger School of Psychiatry affiliated with the Veterans Administration. Some older veterans from World War I were languishing on the back wards. This was not exactly high status placement for staff physicians, couch-bound residents, adjunctive therapy staff, or Freudian researchers. Some basic research dealt with withering dendrites, but there was little interest in studies aimed at improving the quality of life for these long-term older psychiatric patients.

A definitive medical diagnosis requires the specific skills and knowledge of physicians. Another set of skills, knowledge, and attitudes is needed by those responsible for the day-to-day care of an individual exhibiting deteriorating cognitive functioning with all of its subsequent regressive behavior in emotional, social, vocational, and familial aspects of life.

Why reach beyond medical diagnosis? Who will be involved in maintenance, prevention, care of the long-term client? What are the goals of treatment? Why do we need teamwork? How can we keep the patient, staff, and family from burnout? How do we convince the medical profession that maintenance and prevention are as exciting and rewarding as quick, precise technical intervention and cures? How do we sell management that dynamic, long-term care is an integral part of the contiuum of delivery of services?

Dr. James C. Folsom was assigned that mission-impossible in 1958 when he was asked to work with a pilot study in rehabilitation for geriatric mental patients at Winter V.A. Hospital. Staff burnout was the initial problem identified by the head nurse and her associate. Patient inactivity was the other major problem. Under the direction of the unit physician, patients were receiving the best and most advanced physical care, but both patients and staff were stifled by the sterile physical and psychological environment. "The employees of the hospital shunned this ward and had to be forced to accept tours of duty when vacancies occurred. Among the employees, time off for sickness and accidents was high. The general feeling of the whole ward was described aptly by one of the employees as a 'waiting room for Hell.' "[3]

The director and chief of staff had responded to the nurses' request for assistance and followed their suggestion to select Dr. Folsom to direct the study because they needed a prime mover; an enthusiastic patient advocate; a psychiatrist who had the skills, knowledge, and attitudes to employ milieu therapy as the focus of the treatment program; and a Tom Sawyer who could lead staff into painting their fence.

Following the Menninger philosophy that involvement of all staff is vital to decision making in the practice of good psychiatry, Dr. Folsom pushed for organization of a rehabilitation team as the decision making body for promoting change. Team meetings permitted nursing assistants to report their observations of patient behavior to work through their problems with 24-hour care and to begin to recognize their responsibility as members of a milieu treatment team.

Moving from a strict authoritarian medical model of treatment to a team centered management style addressing problems in psychosocial domains is a wide leap across a river full of territory protecting crocodiles, but, with the full support of top management, this rehabilitation team changed a custodial ward into an active rehabilitation unit. There were substantial positive changes with these debilitated patients, but the most surprising change was in the "attitude of the employees."[4] Holden and Woods, in 1982, include "increased morale among those using it" as one of the side-effects of reality orientation.[5]

In addition to the team concept taught by the Menninger School of Psychiatry, two other basic communication devices promoted consistency of staff approach and active patient involvement in treatment. Both attitude therapy and milieu therapy have been an integral part of the development of reality orientation. As Folsom and colleagues refined the process in long-term care settings with meager resources, the three concepts were simplified to adapt to the available staffing resources. For a viable reality orientation program, team approach, attitude therapy, and milieu therapy must be built in or it can deteriorate into a neglected technique relegated to aides and orderlies because of lack of supervisory involvement of the professional and managerial levels.

The name "reality orientation" was created during development of a geriatric program in a state psychiatric hospital in Iowa where a concerned and involved internist was able to adapt and support the concepts under Dr. Folsom's leadership, then chief of staff.

Further development of training programs took place in Tuscaloosa, Alabama, through a centrally funded training program. There were approximately 23,000 interdisciplinary trainees from that program over a 12-year span. Reality orientation as a technique for overcoming confusion (especially with the aged) has become such a widespread part of the long-term care programs within the Veterans Administration system that I was unable to obtain statistics on the incidence or the quality of its use. I have conducted my own observations during visits to 14 medical centers within the last five years. In all of the appropriate units, I saw RO Boards; and staff, when queried, said they "did RO." References to reality orientation are commonplace in the literature pertaining to problems of confusion in the elderly.

To come full circle, the need to include consideration of the environmental, psychological, emotional, familial, educational, vocational, as well as physical problems of aging veterans has moved from one ward to systemwide need. It is time to re-emphasize the cost-effective team approach and milieu therapy aspects of reality orientation; capitalize on the communication system for psychiatric problems offered by attitude therapy; recognize that reality orientation is a management tool; and integrate it into the total rehabilitation evaluation, programming, quality assurance, and tracking systems for long-term care.

Those in the private sector or in private practice may not identify with all this stated need for evaluation and treatment of the "whole" person. In the legal section of *Nursing Homes,* Hirsh reminds us that "Medical care is no longer exclusively delivered by the physician; it is a team effort. The nursing home, or any health institution, now is a health care provider in its own right, and its employees are the physician's teammates. Each is responsible not only for his part, but for the patient as a whole."[6]

Not only is the team necessary in delivery of care, but support and input from other team members may help the physician making the diagnosis. In a study of errors and omissions in diagnostic records on admission of patients to a nursing home, the primary diagnosis was inaccurate with 64% of these 100 patients. With 84%, the secondary diagnoses were either lacking or inaccurate."[7] On the other hand, Loeser and Dickstein found a high degree of diagnostic accuracy on admission to a nursing home. They attributed the discrepancy in these two studies as: "The greater amount of pertinent medical, psychiatric, and social input that can be evaluated, the less likelihood there will be of missed or inaccurate diagnosis. Definite benefits are obtained from thorough and meticulous intake procedures; a full multidisciplinary staff including medical, psychosocial, and psychiatric personnel; and discussion of all the available information."[8]

I emphasize the complexities of geriatric evaluation and care to counteract the belief that reality orientation is a simple technique. It is simple if one already has a fully developed successful team approach to problem identification and solution. It is simple if one has established a well-controlled communication system to promote consistency of approach for psychiatric problems.

It is "simple" if aides and orderlies function as therapeutic rehabilitation team members. It is simple if one has incorporated meaningful activities as part of each individual habilitation plan. It is simple if one has a fully developed continuum of programs to match the continuum of presenting problems. It is simple if staff and family members have been trained and supervisory elements are in place to insure follow-through with implementation of all these concepts.

Even the techniques of this simple treatment approach can be misused. Holden and Woods summarize a warning about the misuse of reality orientation by saying that the "application of the attitudes underlying R.O. is necessary rather than rigid adherence to the methods."[9]

I became concerned at a Miami conference in 1974 when I heard a reality orientation instructor say that one had to have a bowl of plastic fruit to start an RO class, and when a master instructor responded to my suggestion of consideration of transference in an unhealthy situation with nursing aides that she didn't have to know anything about transference because they were not having any trouble with their bus system! Folsom's continuing development of reality orientation through the publication of a pamphlet entitled "Help Begins at Home" shows more emphasis on the whys rather than the hows.[10]

Some of my concern for the easy drift of reality orientation training and implementation toward an isolated "instant cure" was translated into action following work in rehabilitation medicine at the George Washington University School of Medicine. The life skills and subsequent problem-oriented record through life skills grants had been funded to assist with deinstitutionalization at a long-term-care facility for the retarded.[11] Because staff identified the major problem as poor communication, I used the two best communication devices I knew—attitude therapy and team approach. We evaluated all the clients with the adaptive behavior scale, trained the staff in its use; taught them attitude therapy, and broke the staff into maxi- and mini-teams so that direct care personnel and clients would be involved in decision-making.[9]

We incorporated H.E.W. guidelines into the evaluation, programming, and tracking system we developed because the institution with which we were associated for those two grants was under court order. Many of those same quality assurance requirements are designated in the current J.C.A.H. standards. An analysis of the compliance items most often raised during J.C.A.H. surveys within the Veterans Administration shows that this team planning/tracking system covers 100% of the items in the areas of treatment plans, treatment plan review, quality of care, progress notes, and discharge summary. Coverage within the 70 to 80% range includes compliance items for volunteer service, patient care monitoring, social service, and medical service; and for the 60–70% range, nursing, psychiatric care unit, rehabilitation, and intake compliance issues are incorporated in the system.[12]

One major goal of these two projects was to incorporate the problem-oriented medical record system into a generic evaluation/treatment format that could be individualized and used by both institutional and community team members as the client moved through developmentally sequenced levels of care in both institutional and community placement settings. This proved to be an effective training and tracking tool, and helped to avoid fragmentation for the multiproblem population. "For the elderly patient with multiple pathologies and functional deficits, fragmentation of care can adversely affect cost, quality, and outcomes."[13]

We employed the "life skills" format to integrate and summarize the information most pertinent to direct-care staff, family members, or volunteers as they functioned as designated members of the Mini-Team. The first part of this format included a basic working history offering enough pertinent information that even a volunteer could keep communication with a confused patient reality focused. To be sure that inappropriate or nontherapeutic communications between team members and clients were diminished, we used attitude therapy to help team members tighten controls for more consistent feedback to aberrant or self-defeating behaviors. Designation of both maxi- and mini-team members documented roles and responsibilities for both the clients and those involved in the rehabilitation process.

Part of this revision provided a short-cut method to document observations of physical and behavioral problems. This should assist in those situations where physicians do not spend the major portion of their time in direct observation of elderly, multiproblem clients or where psychiatric consultation is infrequent. According to Beard, psychiatric diseases are present in 40% of a nursing home population.[14] To assist in identifying the range of behavioral symptoms exhibited in dementia as well as confusion caused by other physical or psychological problems, a list of symptoms has been added to help differentiate the regressive features of Alzheimer's disease.

In the third part of this team planning/tracking system, reality orientation as the treatment approach to deficits in cognitive functioning is integrated with the other life skills evaluation in ambulation, activities of daily living, communication and socialization, and vocational skills.

Accountability for mini-team involvement in the total evaluation/programming/tracking system gives supervisory personnel a format to monitor and reward direct-care staff or families for use of rehabilitation concepts and programs. The documentation format was developed to focus on both the successes and problems the client experiences in broad life skills areas; implementation of this system, or any system that promotes teamwork; evaluates strengths and problems in life skills; establishes accountability for goal-setting and attainment; is client-centered; structures staff observations in both physical and emotional fields; includes a system for consistent staff communication in dealing with behavior problems; meets most quality assurance requirements for individual rehabilitation planning and tracking; integrates information from the medical record; helps to bridge the gap between diagnosis and direct care; and includes programming for RO should help insure the circle is more nearly closed from conception to practise.

The first book on the subject of this "aspirin" intervention to the problem of confusion, especially among the elderly, was "based on the inspiration of the work of James Folsom and Colleagues in the United States."[15]

In the conclusion of a chapter on the effectiveness of reality orientation, a summary statement of the research indicates there is "some evidence that RO changes patients; in particular, verbal orientation has most often been shown to be improved. The question of generalization to other areas of functioning remains open."[16] In spite of a lack of basic research to support the dramatic changes documented with individual patients, Holden and Woods state: "In the long run it may be at an institutional level that RO makes its most important and far-reaching changes. In order for staff to change in ways consistent with RO the whole ethos of the institution may have to change, and in this light RO may be seen as a philosophy for a dramatic change from purely custodial care to a care that firmly places the emphasis on the needs and potential of the individual."[17]

It was through the Veterans Administration that this "most intensively researched of the psychological approaches to confusion" was developed.[18] Benjamin Wells, former associate chief medical director, said:

> The problem of the senile patient who is confused and disoriented is a large one, and one that exacts an enormous social, economic, and humanistic toll. Reality Orientation is only one of many methods of rehabilitation. Its goals are often modest, but their achievement is a triumph when seen in relation to the drabness of total senility that might have been. "It is better to light one candle than to curse the dark."[19]

That article was written in 1968. The statement is even more pertinent today as we face the demographic imperative and clinical realities of both the aging veteran and the aging public.

REFERENCES

1. Holden, U.P. and Woods, R.T.: *Reality Orientation, Psychological Approaches to the Confused Elderly.* Edinburgh, London, Melbourne and New York, Churchill Livingstone, 1982, pp. 14, 15.
2. Folsom, J.C. and Folsom, G.S.: The real world. *Mental Health:* 29–33, summer 1974.
3. Folsom, J.C.: Reality orientation for the elderly mental patient. *J. Geriatr. Psychiat.:* 294, spring 1968.
4. Ibid, p. 295.
5. Holden and Woods, op. cit., p. 14.
6. Hirsh, H.L.: Duty to stop, look, listen, and communicate. *Nursing Homes:* 37, September/October 1983.
7. Miller, M.B. and Elliott, D.F.: Errors and omissions in diagnostic records on admission of patients to a nursing home. *J. Am. Geriatr. Soc. 34:* 108.
8. Loeser, W.D. and Dickstein, E.S.: Avoiding diagnostic errors in admitting patients to a nursing home. *J. Am. Geriatr. Soc. 27:* 558, 1979.
9. Holden and Woods, op. cit., p. 223.
10. Public Information Office, International Center for the Disabled.
11. Folsom, G.S.: *Life Skills for the Developmentally Disabled. Manual for Trainers.* Washington, D.C. Division of Rehabilitation Medicine. George Washington University, 1975.
12. Folsom, G.S.: *Team Planning/Tracking System.* Unpublished.
13. *DM&S Issues.* January 1983.
14. Beard, W.J., Kalau, E.I., and Noback, R.K.: Geriatric education in a nursing home. *Gerontologist 23:* 133, 1983.
15. Holden and Woods, op. cit., p. 14.
16. Ibid, p. 93.
17. Ibid, p. 94.
18. Ibid. pp. 13, 14.
19. Stephens, L.P.: *Hospital and Community Psychiatry Service. Reality Orientation,* p. 9.

"Who Did You Used to Be?"
The Psychological Process of Aging's Impact on Institutionalization: Implications for Activities

Sally S. Garrigan

Comic strips generally depict a humorous event. Picture now a cartoon with two retired gentlemen seated on a park bench. One turns to the other and asks, "Who did you used to be?" (from *the small society* by Brickman). Brickman's attempt at humor depicts what the psychological process of aging is all about. The question the man poses implies a "life" before retirement, a pre-retirement "person" now lost and gone forever. At retirement age, one is well on their way in the aging process, a process that actually is a lifelong one. For a few years in that process we acquire and gain but for most of that process we lose. LOSS is what the psychological process of aging is all about.

The total self that is a result of those years is made up of many parts. While it is possible to continue growing and there is always room for self-growth, the loss factor gains on us and in fact dominates the process in later years.

At birth the first thing we acquire is a name. During the acquisition years we gain a career or job or some form of accomplishment that we identify with. I *AM* a teacher, I *AM* a lawyer, I *AM* a welder. Many acquire a spouse and thus become half of a commitment. Children join some of us and expand our roles in life. In the process we have established our own homes and surrounded ourselves with personal belongings. We establish a lifestyle related to our economic re-

---

This article was submitted for presentation at the 1984 National Association of Activity Professionals' Conference. Please address inquiries to: PO Box 701, Pierre, SD 57501.

75

sources and health status. A large part of who we are is identified by how we spend our leisure time; what our hobbies are. We now have a picture of a total person made up of a name, job, spouse, children, health, money and hobbies. One last ingredient necessary for functioning in this society is what can be referred to as the "numbers game;" that set of identifying numbers we carry around with us—social security number, telephone number, health insurance number, life insurance policy number, Medicare, Medicaid and zip code.

In the psychological process of aging a progression of loss takes place. The children move along in their own process and leave home; the well known "empty nest syndrome." A loss. We reach that magical age of retirement which is for some a sense of accomplishment but for many a loss of purpose and in fact loss of identity. "Who did you used to be?" A loss. These are the years that retirement income determines life style and for many the next step is "breaking up housekeeping" or perhaps reducing a lifetime of belongings and eight rooms to one. A loss. A lifetime of companionship is now in jeopardy as the years go by and brothers, sisters, parents, friends and most importantly, spouses die. A loss. Declining health in the forms of lost vision, lost dexterity, lost mobility, lost memory function and lost endurance as well as declining financial resources all interfere with recreation. Recreation is those hobbies held up to be the saving grace of the "golden years" of retirement. A loss. This total self is now reduced to name and the "numbers game." All that remains is a name and a number. This incomplete person is very often the profile of the person who is admitted to our long term care facilities.

Long term care facilities, nursing homes, retirement centers or extended care facilities are all institutions and institutionalization of a person can mean the ultimate loss for a person; the loss of choice. The most complete and the mentally healthy person is the one who has control over his or her life and that control is maintained by making choices.

Reaction to loss is fairly universal and predictable. Elisabeth Kübler-Ross in *On Death and Dying* identified the stages of reaction to death as denial, anger, bargaining, depression and acceptance. Death is considered the final loss but it is by no means the only loss to which we react in a predictable manner. Close examination of our reactions to the loss of a job, neighbors and friends due to a move, or temporary ability due to injury reveal that we go through the same stages identified as related to reactions to death. The psychological process of aging and its accompanying losses sends us through the very same steps. The impact of institutionalization makes these stages identifiable in many nursing home admissions. The institutional environment itself reinforces the loss factor by eliminating some choices. The daily decisions of whether or not to get up, what time to arise, whether or not to eat, what to eat, when to eat, whether or not to get dressed, what to wear etc. are sometimes eliminated by necessity of routine and efficiency. The nursing home or retirement center admission is reacting to both losses, the loss from the psychological process of aging and the loss of perceived independence and control by being institutionalized. Activity professionals can identify the stages of reaction in their clients.

Very often a new admission presents us with the denial stage by refusing to bring personal belongings to the center. Verbally, there is denial to fellow residents, "I'm not staying very long," or in being unwilling to start a crafts project, "I won't be here to finish it," or reluctance to join in a social function, "I'm not one of the group here." People can deny the placement even to the point of having their mail forwarded but not officially changing their address, "I don't LIVE here."

Anger is the easiest to spot but often the one misinterpreted. The anger that manifests itself in hitting out at staff and statements about the "terrible" food may really be anger related solely to the loss of independence and decision making. Anger directed at family, "they PUT me here," staff, the facility, and fellow residents or even directed at themselves usually is misguided and in need of being channeled in a more positive direction.

The bargaining stage is not easily identifiable and may not be present in all cases. In fact, not everyone goes through all of the stages or through them in the same progression. Occasionally we find a resident who is hanging on to the hope of returning to independent living by bargaining. "If I could just get SOME strength back in this arm, I can cook again" or "If

I could just master transferring into my chair ALONE, I could go home."

Depression is the stage that the media would have us believe is most prevalent among our institutionalized elderly. It is in fact a major problem among the entire senior population, community based included. Depression may be a reaction to the loss factor related to the psychological process of aging. Activity professionals see it most obviously in non-involved residents, residents who sit and stare out the window or ignore all invitations to participate in activities and refuse to be responsible for their own leisure needs, preferring to sleep.

The final stage in the reaction to loss is that of acceptance. This acceptance of placement and in fact the very acceptance of "who I am" rather than the question "Who did I used to be?" holds the greatest implications for activity programs.

The person who selectively participates in the activity program, assumes responsibility for meeting some leisure needs independently, creates a personal environment of their assigned space, initiates contact and friendships with fellow residents and maintains contact with family and friends in the community is in the stage of acceptance.

Activity professionals and their programs have the potential of assisting people to reach this final stage of acceptance. The element of decision making in an activity program is a powerful factor in overcoming the loss of choice. Well planned and implemented activity programs offer opportunities for self-expression, social involvement, emotional well being and meaningful roles. They can crate a purpose for living, going on, doing more and "being."

The psychological process of aging from a loss perspective presents a negative picture. The process also includes achievements and accomplishments and activity programs that capitalize on those positive aspects can be helpful in preserving a complete person who accepts, adjusts and admits who he or she is rather than asks "Who did I used to be?"

"Sign Language Through Discussion" . . . An Innovative Activity

Fred Greenblatt
Jeffrey Rabinowitz

The title of our program, "Sign Language Through Discussion," is of key importance. Our goals are to educate our residents through discussions helping to increase their awareness of the needs of residents who have speech and/or hearing difficulties. Through these discussions, as well as through the formal class of learning Sign Language, we aim to break down the barriers of fear and prejudice. We hope to create new patterns of communication which will result in a mutual feeling of trust and respect for each other.

Although our class began with a nucleus of four residents, the excitement of learning Sign Language and the ability to communicate with the deaf, has created a renaissance among other residents, adding to the growth of our program. The class is helping foster a new attitude towards the deaf and those with communication difficulties.

"Sign Language Through Discussion" offers advantages for the participant as well as for those with these handicaps. Sign Language is a form of physical and emotional exercise, allowing for an individualized feeling of creative self-expression. It opens a new avenue of communication, which often awakens one's awareness and feelings. The implications of emotional exercise indicate that good signing requires the expression of inner feelings which make a simple gesture become a clear statement. Many participants have exclaimed: "This class makes me feel so alive." We feel this is attributed to the re-awakening of inner feelings required in Sign Language.

Fred Greenblatt, MTRS, is Activities Consultant and Director of Activities at the Jewish Home & Hospital for Aged, Kingsbridge Center, Bronx, NY. Jeffrey Rabinowitz is Activities Leader at the same institution.

Finally, we have found that Sign Language has been instrumental in helping some of our residents overcome emotional and psychological problems associated with a physical handicap such as arthritis. Although, at first, some of our residents felt their arthritic fingers would be an obstacle to successful signing, we have found quite the opposite to be true. Learning to sign, despite the handicap of arthritic fingers and hands, has helped eliminate emotional and psychological restraints, creating a positive self-image and increased self-confidence.

How would you react without the sight of your eyes or without the sound we hear every minute of a normal day? How would you feel if you could not speak or communicate with your friend or neighbor? If these questions are too difficult to answer, try an easier one. How would you, as someone with ALL HIS SENSES, react to someone who cannot hear or cannot speak?

History and experience have taught us that those who do not understand others because of physical, psychological and/or emotional handicaps, become frightened of them. This creates barriers which may include fear, distrust, stereotyping and prejudice.

Experience as an activities director in a large Geriatric Institution has demonstrated that those residents who have minimal physical handicaps, tend to disassociate themselves from residents who have severe hearing, visual or speech impairments, especially deaf mutes. Healthier residents will often avoid contact with this group of people. They have even refused to sit near such residents during a recreation activity.

Behavior and attitudes of many of the healthier residents have reflected their feelings, which on several occasions depict various stereotypes. Very often a mute resident's hearing impairment and inability to speak or communicate becomes associated with someone who has very little intelligence. Thus, the physical handicap creates a barrier which becomes difficult to overcome.

Our activity "Sign Language Through Discussion," has proved to be one of the most meaningful activities we have had at our facility. We are fortunate in having a staff member who knows the language of Signing. It is with my goals and responsibility as Activity Director of The Jewish Home and

Hospital for Aged, Bronx, New York, and his skills, that we have established this worthwhile program.

The aging process has been associated with the decline of one's senses to varying degrees. This deterioration of hearing, eyesight and/or communication often lead to new behavior or social patterns, resulting in increased feelings of isolation. The ability to sign and communicate with others, despite the degeneration of one's senses associated with the aging process, undoubtedly leads to increased self-confidence in the resident participating in the program. The art of Sign Language is one more tool which can be used successfully to help overcome the obstacles of growing old.

Although we realize we are unique in our situation, by having a staff member whose knowledge includes that of signing, we cannot help but emphasize the importance of this activity. Any activity which helps crack the wall of prejudice and respect among those living together and sharing the same community, must be recognized as an activity of special significance.

As an Activity Director, a professional in the field of Gerontology and a concerned human being, it gives me great pleasure to have helped initiate and implement such a worthwhile activity.

They Need Us, We Need Them:
A Study of the Benefits
of Intergenerational Contact

Bonnie B. Lindquist

ABSTRACT. This paper first examines living arrangements for elderly which will facilitate intergenerational contacts with a minimum of energy to be used. Secondly the issue of the need of intergenerational contact on the part of the elderly population is explored. The final segment of the paper tells the story of intergenerational contact in the context of a program given in a home for the elderly. The conclusion of the paper is that intergenerational contact is successful when programs are better attended for the re-call program.

Fifteen years ago a friend and I rehearsed a program of familiar songs, a folk song or two, solos and four community sing selections and we performed for Des Plains Golden Agers and St. Matthew Home in Park Ridge. Why the elderly? A rewarding audience? Surely. Immediate satisfaction? Yes.

When my sister moved to Wisconsin we wanted to sing together. We wanted to engage our audience in the program. We wanted them to give back energy. Thus our programs are in the nature of outreach, an interconnecting of energies. I have seen our audience stimulated for living—going back to their rooms different than when they came into the large room to hear some singing. We have done ten outreach programs in the last year and a half.

As I do more of these outreach programs I have become more interested in the elderly and their problems. I became

Ms. Lindquist is Activities Therapist, St. Matthew's Lutheran Home, Park Ridge, IL. Please address inquiries to: 1321 Willow Avenue, Des Plains, IL 60016.

This article was originally submitted to The National Association of Activity Professionals, for potential presentation at the NAAP 1984 Conference.

interested in the benefits of the contact between generations or age groups for the elderly. So my first task is to explain types of institutions from minimum to maximum care.

Institutions for the elderly run on a continuum of care needed, from little care and some sociability to 24-hour care, supervision, and attention. Day Care Centers for the elderly are available. In Omaha my friend Marj takes her mother, a stroke victim, to a Day Care Center during the hours that Marj works. Her mother is given her medication, a hot midday meal, and sociability. The result is that Marj's mother has the care she needs and the support of intergenerational contact in the evenings and over the weekends.

Day Care Centers can fulfill a variety of needs from the social to the medical for the elderly.[1] Thus a senior can stop in for a portion of the day, during lunchtime for a hearty meal or go on an excursion with the group. For the senior that cannot function alone during the day, there is a place to be that will give the care and supervision needed. In the case of serious physical impairments, the third-level care that is available is the Day Hospital.[2] Day Hospitals give the care that full-time institutions give but allow the person to remain in the community. "Tillie Davis, ill with Parkinson's disease, does well to get herself dressed . . . There is not strength left over for maintenance . . . The day care center keeps her independent."[3]

Hospices allow the very ill person to remain as long in the home before death as possible. A hospice in New Haven is a bright cheerful building where families of the terminally ill patients are welcomed and accommodated.[4] The emphasis is on and will continue to be on health care in the home for the longest time possible.

Day Care Centers, Day Hospitals and Hospices are some alternatives to extended care homes for the elderly. Their existance allows the elderly to remain in their communities, thus avoiding the segregation that is so negative. I use these above examples to show that segregation of the elderly is to be avoided, and that care for the elderly is available outside extended care facilities.

Extended care facilities of nursing homes come in a wide variety of styles, cost, and care given. In 1980 Bruce Vladeck wrote these statistics: "Average nursing home has 75 beds, three-quarters of them are proprietary, 5–10% are operated

by the Government, 3,000 are operated by charitable organizations."[5] Many of the Church Homes or Fraternal Homes
are on a buy-in basis. The resident buys a suite plus pays a
monthly fee. For this outlay, the resident has the security of
lifetime quarters and medical attention. Upon the death of a
resident, the apartment is re-sold. These homes should give
good care and great security to the resident. I understand that
a fraternal home which shall remain nameless will be the
receiver of the resident's estate in order that the resident be
guaranteed lifetime care.

Because Federal and State Medicaid and Medicare funds
reimburse homes for services rendered, the Government
mandates levels of care. Illinois inspects proprietary homes
regularly. In spite of care government regulations, care given
varies greatly from home to home. The cleanliness of the
patients is a good indicator as to how the institution is managed. An institution that is poorly managed will not be interested in having a volunteer outreach for their patients, thus
my knowledge of nursing homes is not well rounded. The
number of wheel-chair patients will also tell what level medical care is provided: in a residence hotel such as Chelsea
House, everyone is mobile, in Americana most patients are in
wheel chairs, in Lutheran Home there is a mix of mobile and
wheel chair or skill level patients.

The typical resident of a nursing home is 80, white, wid-
owed or a spinster, of limited means, and suffering from three
or four chronic ailments.[6] Although this paraphrase specifies
age 80 I am using the age 75 as a break-off age. Sixty-five to
seventy-five is the "young old" and function as they did in
their 60's. At age 75 ailments are present and debilitating
effects of failing faculties are more apparent. Malcolm
Cowley writes that "trees on a hill are no longer maples,
oaks, but merely a blur."[7] Thus Mr. Cowley summarizes a
symptom of the problem of diminishing faculties. The problem of failing eyesight was illustrated graphically to me in
February. At Lutheran Home the activity director handed us
our programs re-typed, using the Orator element which types
twice the height of normal letters. If we expect our audience
to read the words, we will use the large element.

Mr. Cowley addresses sociability of the elderly in this way.
Social horizons are narrowing. Old friends are vanishing and

new ones are hard to find.[8] This aspect of sociability is very difficult to deal with. My father, 75, recites the Masonic Funeral Rites. He sees many of his friends die, and sometimes thinks he is the only survivor. In the newsletter from St. Matthew obituaries are listed in the "with the Lord" column.[9]

Marjorie Shadduck, age 74, says that at 74 one can sense what one will die of.[10] This knowledge has come to her very recently and she will not discuss it because she does not want to give it power over her. Marjorie is working under a deadline to finish writing her family history, the result of twelve years of research. Marjorie's deadline is her departure on a three-week tour of the Middle East. Marjorie's life style is not properly the concern of this study, but we shall hear more of the lady's interests and accomplishments later.

Now as to the accomplishments of people well past the young age, 65–75: old age, 75–85 and up. Alex Comfort has used example after example of contributions to society by the elderly. His bias toward accomplishments of the elderly is a result of his fight, his cause against agism.[11]

Accomplishing elderly and segregated elderly are in the same category but their surroundings are very different. Have residents of nursing homes disengaged because they are segregated or are they segregated because they have disengaged? By disengage I mean pull away from and become less interested in life and people. Is this apparent disengagement just a husbanding of energy? Alex Comfort calls the disengagement theory "sludge language" for being excluded or demeaned and liking it.[12] If the theory is viable it has to be optional.[13] The word optional is not often heard in an institution. Who can say that "Minnie" has disengaged—she may be heartily bored by the project that was designed to keep her busy. She may be thinking of times past when she had control over her life, power which control confers, and status conferred by family or profession or both.

The theory of disengagement, while it has not been disproved, and will receive more research, has thus far not been supported by data.[14] Comfort says disengagement is, ". . . an attribute wished on the newly created old to plaster our guilt and provide a piece of jargon to excuse our conduct. Age-proof people will have none of it".[15]

The opposite meaning of disengagement is engagement.

This word encompasses the many needs of institutionalized elderly, and I will define the particular needs within the area of engagement. There have not been many studies made of the humanistic needs of residents of nursing homes.[16] The medical industry has a problem with people who will not get well.[17] Perhaps sociologists have the same problem. It has to do with the warehousing mentality, and care for the elderly that will not change until this frame of mind changes. My conclusions about the needs of the elderly will be the result of my experiences as a visitor in nursing homes.

Touching and holding is important to the institutionalized elderly, "this dignity spawning touching in public places is too rare in nursing homes."[18] When I reach out to a patient, her eyes first tell me I have her full attention. Then she will grasp my hand and we are engaged, we have made contact with each other. For this lady my reach and her grasp will return dignity of her past function that she has lost in an institution. A few draw away from the touch, but only a small proportion. Even more successful is the athletes' double grasp, very open-handed and not dominating. I have to be very careful that the reach for her hand does not establish my dominance; that my reach will not take away her choice of whether to respond or not. My concern for her personhood is very important. The touch assures us all again that we are okay, it assured us as babies and all through our lives. Why should this assurance of touch be needed by the elderly—it is even more needed than for younger ages.

That the residents have to come to an outreach music program, a craft class, a community sing, a class is very important. Activities play a role in limiting or reversing mental, emotional and physical deterioration.[19] The involved and active elderly survive happier and in less pain than elderly who are not active. Gail Sheehy claims that an elderly "Pathfinder" in a nursing home will care for those more needy than she considers herself.[20] Engagement in other peoples' lives and engagement in activities. I recognize this need for activity in the outreach programs, because we have a reciprocal agreement, and that agreement is that we sing together. Our auditors become performers, and contributors. It is important for the elderly to remain doing for others rather than become passive receivers of friendship and entertainment.[21]

Elderly people need the support of generations other than their own, specifically contact with people other than relatives. "Age segregation interferes with mutual support and socialization between age strata."[22] It is often said that children keep us young. Most of the time that adage is correct. So the young or younger that come into the institution to visit with the elderly revive their interest in life, bring them out of themselves. Most of my research has discussed segregation in terms of living location, the retirement village versus the city apartment or suburban home or condominium. Again, not much research has been done about the effects of segregation upon the institutionalized elderly. The subject would not even arise except for my observations of the effects of Music Outreach. So many of our audience are so happy to see us, and when we move out among the wheel chairs, these people are even more excited. One of the homes we were invited to is properly called an extended care facility—its patients ranged from 20 year olds to the elderly. Some of the old people were more alert and took care of the younger patients. There was no age segregation among the audience. Most of the audience were wheel chair patients, and teenage volunteers came for the evening of our program to bring the patients down and then back up to their rooms. The volunteers down to a man were care giving to their charges, and very human about the project.

The director of Sequoias Retirement Life Care Community is 35 years old. The activity director of Lawrence House is in his early twenties. People ask why are these young people doing this? I say, "why not." Hopefully we have a choice as to whether we will be old, but before we make a choice we will consider the alternative. The elderly can teach the young, and the young can teach the old. The benefits to the young of the wisdom of the elderly are real. Falloux writes: "The old man is the high priest of time past, which does not prevent him from being a seer for the time yet to come."[23] Simon de Beauvoir follows this quote with the observation of amazement that old age is greeted only by contempt.[24] What a waste to segregate people away from the rest of society. So as sorry as we feel for the old folks, we should be sorrowing that we cannot benefit from their experience. We will have to go where they are until we have solved the problem of segregation of the sick, poor, elderly.

Finally there is one more need to add to the list. Is there any reason to believe that the minds of the elderly should not be stimulated, specifically by those of a different generation? For what end our society asks do we need to nurture the minds of the old? To the end that the elderly have a right to the nurture of their minds as any other group has in our society. Simone de Beauvoir writes:

> "Old age exposes the failure of an entire civilization. There is only one solution if old age is not to be an absurd parody of our former life, and that is to go on pursuing ends that give our existence a meaning—devotion to individuals . . . intellectual or creative work."[25]

Classes, concerts, new experiences, all help to lighten the load of failing faculties, a body that will not answer all the commands. Even so the mind is not fettered like its housing; how exciting and stimulating it is to use that mind.

There is a group in California called SAGE or Senior Actualization and Growth Explorations. (SAGE, Claremont Office Park, 41 Tunnel Road, Berkeley, CA 94705, tel. 415-841-9859.[26]) SAGE advocates use of meditation techniques, biofeedback and method exercises such as Yoga and Tai Chi to expand minds and help bodies of the elderly. The founder of SAGE says that these techniques used in nursing homes fight the smell of urine and apathy.[27] Discussion groups in nursing homes are lead by SAGE volunteers, and are frequently intergenerational. A 29 year-old man formed a discussion group and they discussed his birthday and what they all did on their 29th birthdays. Finally the young man went around the circle for a birthday kiss. Each lady was transported to a day when she had a gentleman caller.[28] So residents are asked to respond with their concern, to find the depth of emotion, to explore change rather than just rest and relax. These volunteers ask the questions, and people answer—people who have not been asked questions often enough.[29] SAGE wants to be involved with and by the elderly. While they have a methodology, SAGE staffers say it does not take methodology to see a bright-eyed smile on an old face.[30]

So while SAGE will continue to be that crazy group in Berkeley turning the old people on, funding is a problem which they are working on.[31] Their influence will spread through training of elderly care personnel. Part of their income will come from the sale of these training manuals.

SAGE wants to turn the old folks on to living with discussions, exercise regimens, deep breathing and meditation, to life lived more deeply, more completely, and more healthfully. I conclude that SAGE is a successful program and because it uses volunteers of all generations it is a successful intergenerational contact. I hope they find funding and can continue to increase the number of people they reach.

Intergenerational approaches for young and old are explored in an article by Virginia Fraser and Susan Thornton. The Society for Retired Teachers held a conference in 1975 between high school students and seniors. The result was that seniors realized that students were sensitive to their needs. Students found their stereotype thinking toward the aged changed.[32]

Project Foxfire is about our cultural heritage and how we can protect it.[33] Students interview the aged about their youth and the crafts they practiced. This way crafts and skills can be preserved. Students in Hawaii are building a traditional Hawaiian house.[34] This was deemed a worthy project when it became known that only a handful of Hawaiians knew the procedure and the desired result. When completed, this house will be a community Museum.

In Buffalo, MN, 1979, the Retirement Center of Wright County opened a day care center for children 6 months to 12 years old.[35] The administrator said from day one "it was magic".[36] The atmosphere, the sharing between generations is meant to duplicate the extended family that we read about. The administrator claims kids are taught age stereotyping and in this setting they learn to accept people as they are.[37] It is so successful that Wright Retirement Center won the 1980 Innovation of the Year Award from the American Association for the Aging.

The administrator says "it would be depressing" if the kids were not here.[38] The youngsters lighten the burden of old age for the residents of Wright County Retirement Center. Judging from the picture, the children are entranced.

Contact that works. The smile that creases the wrinkles once more shows the immediate benefit of contact with a person of another generation. This smile, full of character, meaning, kindness, pain, tears, is given in return for a touch and perhaps a song that brought a memory back clearly. The smile tells the person giving time and talent that a gift is being given in return. The gift is so immediate that there is no mistake why it is being given.

The gift of the smiles was the first gift we received as we moved up through our audience and reached out for hands to hold as we sang "I Feel a Song Comin' On." We then asked for audience participation to sing "Over There" and we had it in full measure. Again we moved in through the rest of the singers, urging them in dignity to give their voice. Those who are able do, do so with gusto, those who are not able to give signify their participation with small acknowledgements; a movement of their hands, eye movements following us, a slight turn of the head to follow us as we move.

Midway in our afternoon program we saw that the audience was almost noisy; clapping louder, laughing louder and talking among themselves between songs. This is exactly what we want. Activity, stimulation, movement. One lady sings very loud, another's voice is hardly audible, another hums, another taps the rhythm with one foot. Each member of the audience joins in the activity according to their strength.

As we move through the music "There's a Long, Long Trail," "It Ain't Necessarily So," "Getting to Know You," "Edelweiss," "When the Blue of the Night," we see how each song is affecting our audience. Crosby's song strikes home for most of the audience and though we did not print those words, most everybody sings along "Smiles" for us to sing together, a spiritual called "Two Wings." Then Marjorie plays a Bach piece for piano which gives us time to costume for our funny bit, Madame Catchatory and her faithful (?) accompanist Miss Laughingstock, just off the plane (more likely boat) from a successful tour of the capitals of Europe. The criterion for the costumes is: is it awful enough? Frumpy and floppy hats, gobs of beads, an out-of-date tailored suit, and so on. Miss Laughingstock is the hit of the show. She cheerfully, with zest and total lack of sensitivity steals the show, stops the show, and completely captivates the audience. Finally Madame is able to start to sing "Take Me in Your Arms," a deservedly forgotten song written in 1931. A sample of the lyrics: "like the song of the nightingale," "still the embers of love will be glowing deep in my memory"—need I go on? These deathless lyrics finally lead to Miss Laughingstock's complete sobbing breakdown mid-song of course. Meanwhile the audience is refreshed by this mock-serious silliness which contains just enough sibling rivalry to make the whole scene believable. Finally crashing chords signal the end of this song and bows are repeatedly taken. Our frumpy floppy hats come off and we swing into "Ja Da" to be joined by the audience in a great mood, willing to take a few risks themselves.

Our accompanist Marjorie at 74 maintains her own home in Evanston, does substitute organ playing most of the Sundays she is in the country. She epitomizes involvement and inter-generational contact. Marjorie's causes, interests and compe-tencies are legion. She taught 5th graders to write the music and lyrics to make their own songs. I know, I was there. She was thrilling then, and she has become more thrilling with the years. If she goes to a nursing home, she will help others whom she feels are more needy than she.

In conclusion I let the examples of intergenerational contact stand but must add that on return visits to nursing homes and residence hotels, our audience is always measureably (20 to 30%) larger than the first visit audience. I deem that success.

REFERENCES

1. Bert Kruger Smith, *The Pursuit of Dignity* (Boston: Beacon Press, 1977), p. 24.

2. Ibid.

3. Ibid. p. 25.

4. Tabitha M. Powledge, "Death as an Acceptable Subject," *The New Old: Struggling for Decent Aging*, p. 159.

5. Bruce Vladeck, *Unloving Care the Nursing Home Tragedy* (Basic Books Inc, 1980), p. 8.

6. Ibid. p. 13.

7. Malcolm Cowley, *The View from 80* (New York: Viking Press, 1980), p. 54.

8. Ibid.

9. Newsletter, St. Matthew Lutheran Home, March 1982.

10. Interview with M. Shadduck, retired music teacher, Evanston, IL 2/9/82.

11. Alex Comfort, *A Good Age* (New York: Simon & Shuster, 1976), p. 111.

12. Ibid. p. 65.

13. Ibid.

14. Raymond Kuhlen, "Developmental Changes in Motivation During the Adult Years" in *Relations of Development & Aging* (New York: Arno Press 1980), p. 242.

15. Comfort, p. 65.
16. Robert H. Binstock, Ethel Shanas, (ed.) Handbook of Aging, p. 283.
17. Smith, p. 7.
18. Letter, Cloice Lemon, Activity Dir., River Pines Comm. Center, Stevens Point, WI, 3/3/81.
19. Vladeck, p. 26.
20. Gail Sheehy, *Pathfinders* (New York: Morrow & Co., 1981), p. 254.
21. Smith, p. 48.
22. Matilda White Riley and Joan Waring, "Most Problems of Aging are not Biological, but Social" *The New Old*, p. 64.
23. Simone de Beauvoir, *The Coming of Age* (New York: G. P. Putnam, 1972), p. 203.
24. Ibid.
25. Jack Ossofsky, "Nourishing Minds of the Aging" *New Old*, p. 263.
26. Fraser, Thornton, "An Inventory of Innovative Programs" *New Old*, p. 431.
27. Suzanne Field, "Senior Actualization & Growth Explorations (SAGE)" *New Old*, p. 392.
28. Ibid. p. 393.
29. Ibid. p. 392.
30. Ibid. p. 395.
31. Ibid.
32. Fraser, Thornton, p. 447.
33. Ibid. p. 444.
34. Ibid.
35. Chicago Tribune, 16 Jan. 1982.
36. Ibid.
37. Ibid.
38. Ibid.

BIBLIOGRAPHY

de Beauvoir, Simone. *The Coming of Age*. New York: G. P. Putnam, 1972.
Binstock, Robert H. and Shanas, Ethel, eds. *Handbook of Aging*.
Comfort, Alex. *A Good Age*. New York: Simon & Shuster, 1976.
Cowley, Malcolm. *The View from 80*. New York: Viking Press, 1980.
Gross, Ronald, and Gross, Beatrice, eds. *The New Old: Struggling for Decent Aging*. New York: Anchor Books, 1978.
Sheehy, Gail. *Pathfinders*. New York: William Morrow and Company, Inc., 1981.
Smith, Bert Kruger. *The Pursuit of Dignity New Living Alternatives for the Elderly*. Boston: Beacon Press, 1977.
Vladeck, Bruce C. *Unloving Care The Nursing Home Tragedy*. Twentieth Century Fund Study. Basic Books, Inc. 1980.
Letter, Cloice Lemon, Activity Dir., River Pines Community Center, Stevens Point, WI., March 31, 1981.
Chicago Tribune, 16 January, 1982. Section 1, p. 16.
Personal Interview, Marjorie Shadduck, Retired Music Teacher. Evanston, Il. Feb. 9, 1982.
Newsletter, St. Matthew Lutheran Home, March 1982.
Birren, James E., ed. *Relations of Development & Aging*. New York: Arno Press, 1980.

About the Author

In the mid sixties a friend and I prepared a singing program with the elderly population in mind as the audience. My interest in the elderly began then and so in 1980 when my sister moved from Alaska to Stevens Point, WI we prepared a total of four programs and gave these in nine homes for the elderly in the Chicago area and mid-Wisconsin. Concurrently I was studying for my degree at De Paul University and I explored theories of aging. I received my B.A. in 1982 and left the business world and started to work as an activities therapist at St. Matthew, specializing in music activities. I have created and instituted musical involvement programs here at St. Matthew, also I play the piano, sing, and use music that I create to stimulate residents.

I started piano study in 2nd grade and continued to study at Punahou and then started voice lessons at the University of Hawaii. I have conducted choirs and given voice lessons while I was raising four sons. I plan soon to do consulting work in creation of music programs for homes for the elderly. Also I have prepared a one-woman music show "To Be a Pilgrim" for performance.

So music has run a steady thread through my life, and I most enjoy plying my craft in the setting of the geriatric community.

The Effects of Reminiscing
on the Perceived Control
and Social Relations
of Institutionalized Elderly

Donna E. Schafer
Forrest J. Berghorn
David S. Holmes
Jill S. Quadagno

ABSTRACT. A growing body of literature on reminiscing among the elderly suggests it may have adaptive value and therapeutic benefit for older adults. The present study represents an experimental assessment of the impact of three forms of reminiscence interventions on adjustment measures among a sample of institutionalized elderly. One hundred eighty-five residents of a stratified random sample of 32 nursing homes in eastern Kansas participated in one of the study's three experimental or control conditions. Experimental conditions represented a mix of interactive and structured formats. Analysis of covariance indicates that the interventions constitute a relatively weak treatment when compared with control-group means on dependent variables (social relations, memory, perceived control in life, and life satisfaction). However, the effects on the dependent variables differed according to the type of experimental condition. Reminiscence in discussion-group settings enhanced participants' sense of internal control and their social relations compared with radio broadcasts of reminiscence-oriented programs.

Donna E. Schafer, PhD, is Research Associate at the Gerontology Center, Forrest J. Berghorn, PhD, is Associate Professor of American Studies, David S. Holmes, PhD, is Professor of Psychology, and Jill S. Quadagno, PhD, is Associate Professor of Sociology, all at the University of Kansas, Lawrence, KS 66045.

We would like to acknowledge the financial contribution of the National Endowment for the Humanities to the project (grant #AP-20223-81-1775) from which data for this study were derived.

95

Clinical observations, anecdotal reports, and case studies seem uniformly to indicate that reminiscence activity has great value both for the adaptation of older persons and for clinical insights by case workers, therapists, and physicians (e.g., Kaminsky, 1978; Greene, 1982; Romaniuk, 1983; Butler, 1980–81; LoGerfo, 1980–81). On the other hand, systematic empirical investigations do not provide consistent support for the proposition that reminiscing is adaptive or therapeutic. For example, in studying self-esteem and depression among senior center participants, Perrotta and Meacham (1981–82) find "no support for the view that reminiscing may have therapeutic value for older persons;" and Lieberman and Falk (1971) find that "the adaptive function of reminiscence activity is questionable."

Other studies, however, find at least partial support for the benefits of reminiscing. Hughston and Merriam (1982) find that reminiscing improved the cognitive performance of elderly female "high-rise" dwellers in their sample, but that the performance of males declined. McMahon and Rhudick (1964) find no relationship between the tendency to reminisce and intellectual competency, but find that those who were defined as depressed reminisced less than those who were not depressed. Fallot (1979–80) too finds a relationship between reminiscing and depression in that participation in an experimental reminiscence condition relative to a non-reminiscing condition resulted in decreased self-ratings of depression. Fry (1983) also examines depression, as well as ego strength, relative to individual reminiscence in a community-based elderly sample. Results of that study indicate that reminiscing, particularly under more structured conditions, resulted in significant improvement in the dependent depression and ego strength measures relative to no-treatment control subjects Boylin et al. (1976) find a relationship between frequency of reminiscing and one measure of ego adjustment. They also find that one type of reminiscing was significantly related to ego integrity; this was a "life review," which is described by Butler (1963). This interpretation is reinforced by Coleman (1974) who concludes that "life reviewing" is an adaptive response when accompanied by dissatisfaction with one's past life. These results, however, are at variance with those of Havighurst and Glasser (1972) who conclude that pleasant reminiscence is related to good adjustment and high life satisfaction.

Inconsistent results are at least partially attributable to variations in methodological procedures and to rather dramatic variations in samples, ranging from male residents of a Veterans Administration hospital and domiciliary unit (Boylin et al., 1976) to female residents of a retirement center for nuns (Georgemiller and Maloney, 1984). Only three analyses of the adaptive and therapeutic value of reminiscing used the institutionalized elderly as subjects: the Boylin et al. (1976) all-male sample of 41 veterans; one of three of Lieberman and Falk's (1971) samples (N = 43); and Kiernat's (1979) sample of 23 confused nursing home residents, 21 of whom were female.

Several authors have noted that reminiscence activity has social implications (e.g., Perrotta and Meacham, 1981–82; Marshall, 1974; Pincus, 1970; McMahon and Rhudick, 1964; Hughston and Merriam, 1982). Perrotta and Meacham (1981–82), for example, suggest that "reminiscing, despite the stereotype, is a social activity, i.e., persons who reminisce share their memories with others." Yet, only two of the reminiscence studies reviewed by the authors (Georgemiller and Maloney, 1984; and Kiernat, 1979) employed a group context in which reminiscing was evoked. Neither study found significant support for hypothesized relationships between participation in a group reminiscence intervention and enhanced adjustment even though a fairly sizeable body of literature attests to the benefits of group work with the institutionalized elderly (e.g., Johnson et al., 1982; Ingersoll and Goodman, 1980; Miller and Solomon, (1980); Ebersole, 1978; Saul and Saul, 1974; Malnati and Pastushak, 1980).

The major purpose of the present study is to investigate the adaptive value for a sample of nursing home residents of participating in reminiscence interventions relative to no-treatment control subjects. Interventions have been designed to represent both group and individual reminiscing activities, and, following Fry's (1983) research, to reflect varying degrees of structure in eliciting reminiscence.

METHOD

Sampling

The present sample consists of residents of thirty-two nursing homes in eastern Kansas. It is stratified so that, of the eight homes assigned to each of the study's experimental conditions, one is a large urban facility (100 beds or more), three are small urban facilities (fewer than 99 beds), and four are rural or small town facilities (all with fewer than 99 beds). Thus, it is representative of facilities found in the study area, and all experimental and control groups of facilities are comparable in composition.

Subjects

After assigning facilities to experimental and control conditions, nurisng home staff members were asked to identify 10 to 12 residents whom they felt were mentally and physically capable of participating in the program. That is, participants were expected to be mentally alert, sufficiently ambulatory to leave their rooms, and capable of listening and speaking to others. Included in the study are all residents identified by nursing home staff who agree to participate and to be interviewed, and who are willing to sign an informed-consent form. A total of 185 individuals over the age of sixty participated in one of the study's interventions or the non-treatment control group and were pre- and post-tested. Of these, 26.5 percent were male and 73.5 percent female.

Interventions

Condition 1. Fifty-five subjects participated in this condition. Audio tape selections of National Council on the Aging's (NCOA) Senior Center Humanities Program material ("Self-Discovery Through the Humanities") were played for participants in groups as a catalyst for reminiscing about their experiences of childhood or young adulthood (e.g., school days, the Great Depression, work experiences). Following the playing of the taped selection, group members were invited to compare their experiences with those expressed in the taped excerpt. The discussions were conducted by leaders trained by the researchers to evoke participants' reflections. The use of specific material and an explicit format made this condition a structured group intervention. As was the case for all experimental conditions, sessions lasted for one hour each week for twelve weeks.

Condition 2. Thirty-four subjects participated in this condition. Group discussions were conducted by trained leaders on topics that were identical to those presented in the first condition. However, NCOA materials were not used to prompt reminiscing. In this less structured condition, the discussion leader simply presented the session's topic and invited participants to recall their experiences.

Condition 3. Thirty-nine subjects used the same NCOA selection as those in Condition 1, but they were broadcast via closed-circuit radio to the participating facilities. Following the broadcast of selections, an on-the-air discussion of the material by studio panelists and a phone-in forum took place. Subjects were invited to participate in the discussion by using an in-ward WATTS line. For this condition, facilitators assisted participants who wanted to call and needed help. Thus, reminiscing in Condition 3 could be either oral or silent and represented a more individual, rather than group, activity.

Condition 4. No-treatment Control. Fifty-seven individuals were assigned to the control group and were pre- and post-tested at the same intervals as individuals in the three experimental conditions. They were informed that they could participate in a reminiscence discussion program after twelve weeks' time.

Hypotheses

Hypothesis 1. Having experienced the reminiscence intervention in some form, all three experimental groups would "improve" relative to the no-treatment control group on outcome variables indicating adjustment to old age and the exigencies of the institutional environment.

Hypothesis 2. There would be a ranking among the experimental and control groups in terms of degree of benefit derived from program participation. The order of "improvement" from pre- to post-testing would be related to the degree of structure in the condition's format and the extent of social interaction involved: i.e., NCOA tape cassette discussion condition, non-NCOA discussion condition, radio broadcast condition, no-treatment control condition.

Measures

Two interview schedules were developed for this study. One was the instrument administered to residents both before and after participation. The other was given to nursing home staff members (usually Activity Directors) acquainted with the prospective participants. The study includes 13 "background" variables, 8 of which are demographic and 5 of which pertain to conditions in the home. These variables are considered to be independent; that is, not likely to be affected by participation in one of the experimental interventions. The principal function of this set of variables is to test for compositional differences among the 4 conditions. They include sex, race, age, rural-urban residence, schooling, prior living arrangements, marital status, occupation, type of nursing home, number of health problems, tenure in facility, participation in decision to enter the home, and frequency of visits from outside the home.

Fourteen variables are employed to test the effectiveness of the interventions, 8 of which are attitudinal, 4 of which measure social interaction and activity, and 2 of which measure memory. These variables may be considered indicators of adjustment to conditions in the nursing home.

Attitudinal Variables

Two measures of life satisfaction are included in the study. One is an eleven-item derivative of the twenty-item Life Satisfaction Index (Neugarten et al., 1961), which is considered to be multidimensional. Nine of the 20 items produced no variation in responses from the institutionalized subjects in our pilot study and were, therefore, omitted from the present study (range 0–22, M = 12.2 and SD = 5.2). The other is a Cantril ladder (Cantril, 1965) which is a global self-anchoring measure (range 1–9, M = 5.7 and SD = 2.4). Cantril ladders were also used to assess subjects' perceptions of the friendliness of other residents in their facility (range 1–9, M = 6.8; SD = 2.0) and their perception of their own health (range 1–9, M = 6.5; SD = 1.99). Two value measures are included, one regarding life in general and the other regarding life in the nursing home. Both questions were designed to elicit a respondent's strongest value orientation from among: community involvement (including in the latter case the nursing home's activities as a form of community involvement); family relations, friendship; and independence, or getting along as best as one can for oneself. Two control measures were generated, one relating to whether residents felt they had control over things that happened in their daily lives (range 0–2, M = 1.3, SD = 0.9), and the other to whether life in general is controlled by luck, fate, or powerful others (range 0–2, M = 1.5, SD = 0.8).

Social Interaction and Activity Variables

Respondents were read a list of names of other people in the facility also planning to participate in the particular intervention (or control group) and were asked whether or not they knew any of these individuals (range 1–2, M = 1.9; SD = .28) and, if so, how many they knew (M = 4.9; SD = 3.7). A variable was then computed that expressed the ratio between the number of people a respondent knew and the number appearing on that list. The median for this computed variable fell between "1" and "2." Another variable was created to reflect the nature of a person's interaction with the facility's other residents. Responses were coded to reflect the degree of spontaneous activities initiated by the resident (range 1–3, M = 1.9; SD = 0.7). Residents were asked whether there was someone in whom they could confide. A value of "0" or "1" was assigned depending on whether or not a confidant(e) was identified (M = 0.8; SD = 0.4).

Memory

Two measures of memory were generated for the study. A short-term memory measure was based on recall of a list of 19 common words. Scores were assigned on the basis of the number of correct words repeated by the subject (range 0–19,

M = 3.2; SD = 2.1). Respondents also were asked to recall three major historical events—the bombing of Pearl Harbor, assassination of President Kennedy, and Watergate. The more information they could recall about each event, the higher their score (range 0–15, M = 5.4, SD = 3.3).

Statistical Procedures

Two principal statistical procedures were employed. One analysis determined whether there were compositional differences in the treatment and control groups that might have affected the manner in which participants experienced the various reminiscence interventions. Independent variables (listed above) were examined in relation to experimental group membership using chi square for categorical variables and analysis of variance for continuous variables.

Secondly, analyses of covariance were used to examine the differential impact of various interventions on the attitudes, memory, and social relations of participants. In those analyses, the pre-measure served as the covariate, and this procedure eliminated any potential effect of initial differences. Following the analysis of covariance, the Newman-Keuls post-hoc test with studentized range statistic was computed to identify group means that are significantly different from each other within the set of adjusted group means for a given dependent variable produced by the analysis of covariance procedure.

RESULTS

Group Compositional Characteristics

Only two statistically significant relationships were found between background characteristics and experimental group membership. A significant relationship was found between experimental group membership and participation in the decision to enter an institution (x^2 = 23.45, df = 12, p = .02). In this case, Radio Broadcast and Control group subjects were somewhat less likely to have been active participants in the decision to enter an institution than members of the two discussion conditions. Blacks were disproportionately assigned to the Radio Broadcast condition ($x^2 = 25.91$, df = 3, p < .001). As a result of the sampling technique that assigned facilities to experimental conditions, one large urban facility containing a high concentration of black residents was randomly-assigned to the Broadcast condition. Thus, while only 14 of the 185 participants in the study were black, 10 of those were in the Radio Broadcast condition (28 other subjects in this condition were white). An analysis of variance was conducted on the Radio Broadcast condition alone to determine if there were differences between blacks and whites on the six outcome variables significantly related to the experimental conditions (analysis of covariance presented below). Only one, the Cantril ladder life satisfaction variable, was significantly affected by race. Blacks were significantly lower on this measure (F = 8.7, p = .005). While these compositional differences should be kept in mind in regard to the Cantril life satisfaction results, it generally can be concluded that compositional differences among the four conditions were minimal, and that relationships between interventions and outcome variables are not likely to have been a function of demographics.

Impact of Experimental Interventions on Adjustment Measures

The analyses of covariance that were conducted to identify the effects of the interventions revealed significant differences among conditions on 6 of the 14 variables that were considered. The results are summarized in Table 1.

The variables in Table 1 can be grouped in terms of social interaction, feelings of control, and life satisfaction. With regard to social interaction, the findings indicate that participation in the non-NCOA Discussion condition resulted in subjects knowing significantly more residents of the nursing homes than was the case for subjects in any other condition. Related to that is the finding that subjects in the NCOA and non-NCOA Discussion conditions had the highest scores on interaction quality (spontaneous initiation of activities with other residents), but only subjects in the non-NCOA condition had scores that were significantly higher than those of

Table 1: Analysis of Covariance by Experimental Condition

| VARIABLE | ADJUSTED GROUP MEANS | | | | PROBABILITY |
	NCOA DISCUSSION (N)	NON-NCOA DISCUSSION (N)	RADIO BROADCAST (N)	CONTROL (N)	
Ratio: # People Know/List	$.48_a$ (54)	$.66_b$ (34)	$.54_a$ (34)	$.50_a$ (57)	.02
Interaction Quality	2.15_{ab} (54)	2.32_b (34)	1.96_a (38)	1.90_a (57)	.02
Cantril Ladder -Friendliness	7.10_b (50)	7.18_b (29)	5.88_a (33)	6.72_b (38)	.02
Control – Daily Life	1.73_b (55)	1.49_b (34)	1.03_a (39)	1.54_b (57)	.00
Control – Life in General	1.66_b (55)	1.60_{ab} (34)	1.24_a (39)	1.56_{ab} (57)	.04
Cantril Ladder -Life Satisfaction	6.42_{ab} (50)	6.36_{ab} (32)	5.59_a (37)	6.94_b (48)	.02

For each dependent variable, means that do not share a subscript differ from each other at the $p < .05$ level. (Post hoc analysis using Newman-Keuls test) subjects in the Broadcast and Control conditions. Finally, the analysis of the friendliness ratings indicated that subjects in the Broadcast condition perceived other residents as significantly less friendly than did subjects in any of the other conditions. Overall then, it appears that discussion groups (whether using NCOA materials or not) enhanced subjects' interaction with other residents, whereas simply listening to the broadcast with other persons increased subjects' feelings of distance from others.

With regard to feelings of control, on both measures the subjects in the Broadcast condition had the lowest scores. On the Daily Life measure of control the subjects in the Broadcast condition had scores that were significantly lower than those of subjects in every other condition. On the general measure of control, the scores of the subjects in the Broadcast condition were significantly lower than those of subjects in the NCOA Discussion condition. It is clear, then, that participating in the Broadcast condition resulted in lower levels of perceived control.

The measure derived from the LSI-A was not significant across the conditions, while the Cantril ladder measure of life satisfaction was significant. However, its significance was due only to the lower score of the Broadcast condition relative to the Control group.

DISCUSSION

Only limited support has been found for our hypotheses. Two of the three experimental conditions could be said to bring about some improvement on a few adjustment measures relative to the no-treatment control group (Hypothesis 1). In addition, the order in which the experimental interventions were hypothesized to bring out improvement (Hypothesis 2) was only partially confirmed. The two discussion conditions were clearly most beneficial, but the NCOA Discussion condition was not more beneficial than the non-NCOA Discussion condition. The Broadcast condition did not improve levels of adjustment. Indeed, it appears to have been counterproductive.

One conclusion that emerges from this study is that the

experimental reminiscence intervention, in any of its forms, was a relatively weak treatment. The fact that some changes from pre- to post-testing did occur, and for the Control group as well, probably reflects, at least in part, the lack of mental nourishment generally experienced by mentally-alert residents in nursing home environments. Control group participants were simply interviewed twice, amounting to something less than two hours of interaction over a three-month period. Practice effects do not reasonably account for the improvement on Control group scores from pre- to post-testing. Therefore, the only way to explain the improvement on adjustment measures for Control group subjects involves the anticipation of a new and pleasurable experience and, probably, feeling part of a group receiving "special" attention. Given an environment that, at best, is characterized by predictable daily routine, a new experience or even the anticipation of a new experience can be beneficial for those who are mentally engaged and alert. Other studies (McCormack and Whitehead, 1981; McClannahan and Risley, 1975) also have demonstrated that comparatively slight interventions can enhance engagement levels of nursing home residents. The other side of the coin, of course, is that a similarly slight intervention, such as represented by the Radio Broadcast condition, had an adverse effect. Taken together, these results suggest that mentally-alert nursing home residents may be rather susceptible, either positively or negatively, to the effects of interventions. Since there is little in the literature to suggest that a more individual, or silent, reminiscing activity is harmful (although authors disagree about whether or not it is helpful), it does not seem warranted to attribute these results solely to the type of reminiscing evoked. To explain these results, it seems appropriate to examine the manner in which the Broadcast condition was conducted.

Two explanations seem most compelling. First, a broadcast program, even with a phone-in option, is not as flexible and responsive to participants' interests in pursuing one aspect of the topic as opposed to others, as would be the case in an on-site discussion group. In a relatively small discussion group (six to ten participants), there is opportunity for each individual to be heard and have some impact on the course of the discussion, if they choose to do so. In the Broadcast condition, however, if subjects chose to make a call (or asked the facilitator to place a call), they would necessarily have had to compete for time with all other members of that condition (N = 34).

The opportunity to make choices and a sense of control are significantly related to measures of well-being among various populations of older people (e.g., Langer and Rodin, 1976; Campbell, 1981; Berghorn and Schafer, 1981; Mancini, 1980–81; Ziegler and Reid, 1983; Morganti et. al., 1980; Harel and Noelker, 1982). It seems plausible to argue that the comparatively less interactive format imposed by the Broadcast intervention and the greater personal effort required for active participation undermined subjects' sense of control over the program. For the Radio Broadcast intervention, means of the two "control" variables and the Cantril life satisfaction measure dropped from 1.33 to 1.03, 1.44 to 1.23, and 5.89 to 5.57 respectively, while means for the other two interventions and the Control condition increased. These results are consistent with results of other investigations (Miller and Solomon, 1980; Saul and Saul, 1974) that underscore the importance of participants' feelings of control in developing beneficial activity interventions, and enhancing life satisfaction.

There are several reasons why the discussion-group format is likely to enhance a resident's sense of personal control. Whether or not a person previously has been a member of a formal discussion group, virtually everyone has had the experience of talking in small groups. Therefore, such an intervention would not be entirely unfamiliar. The subject of the discussions is, in effect, each person's own life, about which he/she is an expert. Therefore, the resident's status in the discussion group is at least on an equal level with the staff member (discussion leader), a situation that rarely occurs in other areas of nursing home life. Finally, the staff member is able to experience residents as competent individuals.

In contrast, most participants in the Broadcast condition would not have had previous experience calling into a radio program and talking on the air, which means that a stressful situation inadvertently may have been created for participants. As Lawton and Nahemow (1973) point out in their ecological model of aging, if the individual has fairly low competency (or some impairment in functioning) and finds him/herself in an environment (or stressful situation) that poses problems the individual cannot overcome, then "negative affect" or maladaptive behavior results. Therefore, in designing reminiscence or other interventions for institutionalized elderly, practitioners should keep in mind the relationship between individual competence and the demands of a given activity.

CONCLUSION

While the effect of a reminiscence discussion group experience on social relations was modestly beneficial, the effect of a radio broadcast of reminiscence-inducing material was decidedly detrimental to subjects' perceptions of the friendliness of other residents and to their own sense of control, as well as to their life satisfaction. These latter results suggest that practitioners who introduce interventions into long-term care facilities should exercise caution in their design. Although adverse effects can occur if the demands of the activity exceed the capacities of nursing home residents, interventions that do not sufficiently challenge participants to remain intellectually engaged are also unlikely to be beneficial.

A number of rather dramatic anecdotal reports and clinical observations were gathered during the three-month intervention period. Some individuals in the discussion interventions overcame symptoms of social withdrawal and clinically diagnosed depression and became observably more active in the facility's other activities. Other investigators attempting a group reminiscence intervention (Georgemiller and Maloney, 1984; Kiernat, 1979) have observed the same phenomenon; that is, some rather dramatic individual successes but comparatively slight statistical changes from pre- to post-testing. Given that anecdotal reports focus on the exceptional while statistical analyses are based on central tendency, it is not inconsistent to have individual transformations of some note, while at the same time having group results that are not noteworthy. Generally, studies of group interventions attempt to answer the question: What effect does the intervention have on some outcome variable or variables among all members of an experimental group or groups relative to a control group? That was, of course, the general question posed in the present study. A less frequently asked, but equally important question is: What are the characteristics of people who are most affected by the intervention(s) compared with those least affected on some outcome measure or measures? In addition to its intrinsic gerontological and clinical interest, research that attempts to identify such characteristics should prove extremely helpful to therapists and others in designing meaningful activities for residents of long-term care facilities.

REFERENCES

Berghorn, F., Schafer, D. The quality of life and older people. In F. Berghorn, D. Schafer & Associates, *The dynamics of aging.* Boulder, Colo.: Westview Press, 1981.
Boylin, W., Gordon, S., & Nehrke, M. Reminiscing and ego integrity in institutionalized elderly males. *The Gerontologist,* 1976, *16,* pp. 118–124.
Butler, R. The life review: An interpretation of reminiscence in the aged. *Psychiatry,* 1963, *26,* pp. 65–76.
Butler, R. The life review: An unrecognized bonanza. *International Journal of Aging and Human Development,* 1980–81, *12,* pp. 35–38.
Campbell, D. Microenvironments of the elderly. In F. Berghorn, D. Schafer & Associates, *The dynamics of aging.* Boulder, Colo.: Westview Press, 1981.
Cantril, H. *The pattern of human concerns.* New Brunswick, N.J.: Rutgers Univ. Press, 1965.
Coleman, P. Measuring reminiscence characteristics from conversation as adaptive features of old age. *International Journal of Aging and Human Development,* 1974, *5,* pp. 281–294.
Ebersole, P. Establishing reminiscing groups. In I. Burnside, *Working with the elderly: Group process and techniques.* North Scitnate, Mass.: Duxbury Press, 1978.
Fallot, R. The impact on mood of verbal reminiscing in later adulthood. *International Journal of Aging and Human Development,* 1979–80, *10*(4), pp. 348–400.
Fry, P. Structured and unstructured reminiscence training and depression among the elderly. *Clinical Geronotologist,* 1983, *1,* pp. 15–37.
Georgemiller, R., & Maloney, H. Group life review and denial of death. *Clinical Gerontologist,* 1984, *2,* pp. 37–49.
Greene, R. Life review: A technique for clarifying family roles in adulthood. *Clinical Gerontologist,* 1982, *1*(2), pp. 49–67.
Harel, Z., & Noelker, L. Social integration, health and choice: Their impact on the well-being of institutionalized aged. *Research on Aging,* 1982, *4*(1), pp. 97–111.
Havighurst, R., & Glasser, R. An exploratory study of reminiscence. *Journal of Gerontology,* 1972, *27,* pp. 245–253.
Hughston, G., & Merriam, S. Reminiscence: A nonformal technique for improving cognitive functioning in the aged. *International Journal of Aging and Human Development,* 1982, *15,* pp. 139–149.
Ingersoll, B., & Goodman, L. History comes alive: Facilitating reminiscence in a group of institutionalized elderly. *Journal of Gerontological Social Work,* 1980, *2*(4), pp. 305–319.
Johnson, D., Sandel, S., & Margolis, M. Principles of group treatment in a nursing home. *The Journal of Long Term Care Administration,* 1982, *10*(4), pp. 19–24.

Kaminsky, M. Pictures from the past: The use of reminiscence in casework with the elderly. *Journal of Gerontological Social Work*, 1978, *1*(1), pp. 19–31.

Kiernat, J. The use of life review activity with confused nursing home residents. *The American Journal of Occupational Therapy*, 1979, *33*, pp. 306–310.

Langer, E., & Rodin, J. The effects of choice and enhanced personal responsibility for the aged. *Journal of Personality and Social Psychology*, 1976, *34*, pp. 191–198.

Lawton, M. P., & Nahemow, L. Ecology and the aging process. In C. Eisdorfer & M. P. Lawton (eds.), *The psychology of adult development and aging*. Washington, D.C.: American Psychological Association, 1973.

Lieberman, M., & Falk, J. The remembered past as a source of data for research on the life cycle. *Human Development*, 1971, *14*, pp. 132–141.

LoGerfo, M. Three ways of reminiscence in theory and practice. *International Journal of Aging and Human Development*, 1980–81, *12*, pp. 39–48.

McClannahan, L., & Risley, T. Design of living environments for nursing home residents: Increasing participation in recreation activities. *Journal of Applied Behavioral Analysis*, 1975, *8*, pp. 261–268.

McCormack, D., & Whitehead, A. The effect of providing recreational activities on the engagement level of long-stay geriatric patients. *Age and Ageing*, 1981, *10*, pp. 287–291.

McMahon, A., & Rhudick, P. Reminiscing in the aged: An adaptational response. *Archives of General Psychiatry*, 1964, *10*, pp. 292–298.

Malnati, R., & Pastushak, R. Conducting group practica with the aged. *Psychotherapy: Theory, Research and Practice*, 1980, *17*, pp. 352–360.

Mancini, J. Effects of health and income on control orientation and life satisfaction among aged public housing residents. *International Journal of Aging and Human Development*, 1980–81, *12*(3), pp. 215–220.

Marshall, V. *The life review as a social process*. Paper presented at the Annual Scientific Meeting of the Gerontological Society, Portland, Ore., October, 1974.

Miller, I., & Solomon, R. The development of group services for the elderly. *Journal of Gerontological Social Work*, 1980, *2*(3), pp. 241–257.

Morganti, J., Nehrke, M., & Hulicka, I. Resident and staff perceptions of latitude of choice in elderly institutionalized men. *Experimental Aging Research*, 1980, *6*, pp. 367–384.

Neugarten, B., Havighurst, R., & Tobin, S. The measurement of life satisfaction. *Journal of Gerontology*, 1961, *16*, pp. 134–143.

Perrotta, P., & Meacham, J. Can a reminiscing intervention alter depression and self-esteem? *International Journal of Aging and Human Development*, 1981–1982, *14*(1), pp. 23–30.

Pincus, A. Reminiscence in aging and its implications for social work practice. *Social Work*, 1970, *15*(3), pp. 47–53.

Romaniuk, M. The application of reminiscing to the clinical interview. *Clinical Gerontologist*, 1983, *1*(3), pp. 39–43.

Saul, S. R., & Saul, S. Group psychotherapy in a proprietary nursing home. *The Gerontologist*, 1974, *14*, pp. 446–450.

Ziegler, M., & Reid, D. Correlates of changes in desired control scores and in life satisfaction scores among elderly persons. *International Journal of Aging and Human Development*, 1983, *16*(2), pp. 135–146.

The Design and Implementation of Memory Improvement Classes in the Adult Day Care Setting

Evelyn Capuano

ABSTRACT. A prevalent fear of elderly people concerns the loss of one's memory and the implication such an impairment creates. This article describes memory improvement classes which significantly enhance memory functions in a heterogeneous group of elderly individuals in the Adult Day Care setting. The group is comprised of people with varying degrees of cognitive function from those with severe, irreversible memory loss to individuals whose memory functions are still intact.

INTRODUCTION

Memory lapses occur in people of all ages. In general, however, the degree of significance attached to such lapses differs with the age of the individual involved. Young and middle-aged people who forget something are usually unconcerned. Older people who experience memory lapses, however, all too often become embarrassed and afraid they are losing their minds.

THE DECISION TO ADDRESS THE ISSUE

Precisely because memory lapses create emotional distress in older people there is a tendency to avoid discussing the phenomena. However, recent findings, ours and others, suggest that memory improvement strategies can be learned, and

Evelyn Capuano, RN, MS is the director of Adult Day Care, Waveny Care Center, 3 Farm Road, New Canaan, CT 06840.

that willingness to openly discuss memory impairment with older people can, in fact, substantially decrease their often overwhelming anxiety about the subject (Wilson et al., 1984).

This author's invitation to adult day care clients to participate in exercises through which "we will learn ways to bring about memory improvement in ourselves" was received enthusiastically.

BEHAVIORAL OBJECTIVES

The objectives which were set for the memory improvement classes at the start were as follows:

1. The classes should be fun.
2. The classes should be stress-free.
3. Participants should experience immediate success.
4. Participants should be able to transfer knowledge learned in class to every day living.
5. Classes should provide a forum in which participants could discuss their own anxieties and fears which often evolve from memory impairment or anticipated memory impairment in the future.
6. Classes should provide the opportunity for participants to share their own successful strategies to cope with memory impairment.

THE DESIGN AND IMPLEMENTATION OF CLASSES

Classes described herein are based on the paradigm of Garfunkel and Landau but have been altered significantly to meet specific needs of day care clients with varied levels of memory capabilities.

Garfunkel et al. describe the importance of educating participants concerning the three main reasons for memory impairment which are stress, inattention and depression and the three most effective memory aids, concentration, repetition and association (Garfunkel et al., 1981).

We have chosen to begin each class by reviewing these

points. An effective strategy is to use a poster board which, on one side, lists Memory's Enemies: stress, inattention and depression and on the reverse side, Memory Aids: concentration, repetition and association. Amusing sketches of faces which represent stress, inattention and depression as well as concentration, repetition and association provide a light-hearted touch.

SHARING EXPERIENCES

A technique which is effective in encouraging participation is to ask each one present to mention something which he/she finds difficult to remember. Answers may include forgetting to take one's medications, forgetting to water the plants or forgetting to turn off the stove. All responses can be listed on a chalk board. From this list, participants can be asked to select those items which are essential to remember and those which are simply nice to remember. The list of items essential to remember is always far shorter than the list of items which are merely nice to remember. The obvious conclusion one must draw is, not everything has to be remembered.

Another helpful strategy is to encourage participants to share particular techniques which each uses to remember what is essential to remember. The responses in our group included putting a shoe on the kitchen table, which reminded one man to take his shoes to the cobbler, a woman volunteered that putting her pill in a saucer near the bathroom sink at bedtime reminded her to take the pill each morning. A staff member said she is able to remember to mail letters if she puts them on top of her briefcase the night before.

PROVIDING MEMORY TASKS

A means by which participants can learn to apply memory improvement strategies is to assign each a specific memory task to complete during the course of each class. Our findings suggest the following technique is successful. The leader begins by giving these instructions to the group:

1. I will whisper something to each one of you which I would like you to try to remember. Listen carefully to what I've said. If you haven't heard me, stop and ask me to repeat it, do that as often as necessary.
2. Repeat it to yourself three times.
3. Make an association between what I ask you to remember and something you already know.
4. I will later ask you to repeat what I said. If you can do so, that's great. If you are unable to do so, say "so what!" You will do better next time.

The specific task can then be given to each individual. A concise message is "Please try to remember＿＿＿＿＿. Got it?" Each participant nods affirmatively when he/she hears and understands the assignment. Immediately after each subject states what he was asked to remember, it is helpful to reward the performance through the use of such terms as "good," "great," "very nice." Using exactly the same technique, tasks in various categories may be given as follows: colors (two then three at a time), names of people, telephone numbers, phrases, sentences, several unrelated items on a shopping list, errands to make.

THE IMPORTANCE OF IMAGERY

A very valuable component of memory training involves the use of imagery. Class participants can be taught the technique of creating a mental image by being instructed to "paint a picture in your head of what you want to remember." For example: three unrelated items on a shopping list can be recalled by imagining how they will be used. A retired journalist described how he was able to recall razor blades, carbon paper and ice cream: "I simply pictured myself sitting at the typewriter, late at night, when I needed a shave. I ran out of carbon paper so I had to stop writing. As a reward to myself for working so late I had a huge dish of strawberry ice cream."

To remember errands one needs to do, it is helpful, again, to devise a mental image. Trips to the library, post office, dentist and barber shop can be easily recalled if one pictures going into each building for a particular purpose. In this situation it is helpful to weave the information into a story. One technique might involve picturing oneself walking through the library door to get a book of stamps to take to the post office. While at the post office one meets his dentist who says "After I fill your tooth I'm going to get a haircut." The more unusual the plot of such a story is, the easier it will be to remember.

MODIFICATION FOR MEMORY IMPAIRED INDIVIDUALS

As earlier stated here, this group includes several individuals who have severe, irreversible short-term memory impairment. With these individuals a different approach is necessary. First, the task which is asigned should be something familiar to them. A retired handbag salesman was asked to remember the sentence "Handbags are a big business." A former resident of the Bronx, New York, is asked to remember "The Yankees play in the Bronx." In addition, memory impaired individuals are given their assignment last and are asked to repeat it first.

With all of the subjects, a concerted effort is made to avoid any interruption of thought between the time of assignment and the point at which it is to be repeated. To that end, group members are careful to maintain silence while the process is being conducted.

With all participants an important factor seems to be the wish to experience success. In this way the cycle of stress—memory impairment—can be broken.

SUMMARY

This activity is not designed with regard to strict scientific discipline but it is effective. In summary, the following statements can be made about it:

1. Participants enjoy the activity and, indeed, when it is not conducted they express disappointment.
2. In the three-year period during which the classes have been conducted, most participants report memory improvement as a direct result of the activity.

3. Anxiety about memory loss is diminished among members of the group.
4. This group of individuals who have worked together to improve memory has become more cohesive as a direct result of the shared experience.

REFERENCES

Garfunkel, Florence, et al. A memory retention course for the aged. Washington. D.C. The National Council on the Aging, 1981.

Swilop, Sana. How to improve your memory. Discover. November 1983. p. 28.

Wilson, Barbara, et al. Clinical Management of Memory Problems. Rockville. Maryland: Aspen Systems Corporation, 1984.

The Effects
of Pet Facilitative Therapy
on Patients and Staff
in an Adult Day Care Center

Joanne Damon
Rita May

This study focuses on adult day care and the effect of pet facilitated intervention on individuals isolated by dementing illness. Despite an abundance of anecdotal evidence that supports the value of employing pets for therapeutic purposes, only 3 controlled investigations in this area have been reported to date. While the authors are only able to contribute anecdotal observations at this time, we believe this evidence continues to support the therepeutic contribution that pets can make to participants in an adult day care center. In the absence of clear evidence of the effects of pet-human interactions, administrators of health care facilities act on the basis of intuition and personal experience.

Adult day care can be seen as a prevention strategy allowing a frail, at-risk elderly person to remain in the home and living with family despite physical or mental handicaps. Because many of individuals appropriate for such a setting, which provides not only support but respite for family members, are in the early stages of Alzheimer's disease or moderately impaired from multi-infarct dementia, the addition of pets to such a setting through a visitation program seemed of interest. Adult day care provides 5–6 hours of quality supervision for the confused aged, thus giving familial care-givers a respite, freeing them to work or enabling them time to ac-

Ms. Damon, RN, MEd., is Assistant Professor, School of Nursing, University of North Carolina, Chapel Hill, NC 27514. Ms. May, BA, is Coordinator, Community Life Program, Durham, NC.

complish other tasks. One such program exists at the Community Life Center, which is housed in the Duke Memorial Methodist Church, Durham, NC. The Community Life Program is designed to provide for the needs of the frail population, with a focus on independence, wellness, and maintenance for the individual enrolled. The primary goals are to prevent inappropriate institutionalization and to provide family respite.

The clients who attend this day care center are the elderly with mental and/or physical disorders; senile dementia (at the time of this study 7 to 30 participants were diagnosed as having Alzheimer's disease), strokes with varying degrees of impairment; visual disturbances; and the majority of participants have impaired communication skills. While new members have joined the group in the last two years, the majority of the participants have remained. Several participants have not participated in activities or communicated with any other member of the group nor with staff members during this period. Because the group is very large and diverse in terms of needs, the coordinator finds general programming complicated as a great variety of activities must be considered. A concern of the coordinator based on 2 years observations of both participants and non-professional staff is that the activities selected must facilitate greater interaction of staff with the uncommunicative clients.

The investigators have followed current literature in order to generate ideas about programs that would benefit the uncommunicative participant and encourage greater interaction between the non-professional staff (and professional staff also) and these "silent" participants. One most notable study by Robb (1979) conducted at the Veteran's Administration Medical Center in Pittsburgh, PA studied the effectiveness of "A Wine Bottle, A Plant, and a Puppy" as catalysts for social behavior. Of these three stimuli, the puppy produced the most dramatic increase in social behavior. This effect is not surprising since a puppy offers love and unconditional acceptance in addition to stimulating multiple senses, smell, touch, vision, and hearing. Robb (1981) also noted that the staff interacted more with those participants who were positively affected by their interactions with pets (smiling behavior, conversing with pets as well as others nearby).

Another study of particular interest was an experimental study conducted by Francis and Turner (1982) in which they introduced 8 puppies to residents at the "experimental" home for three hours once a week for 8 weeks. The residents in the Control group had weekly human visitors only. Each group was pre and post-tested for eight variables: health self-concept, life satisfaction, psychological well-being, social competence and interest, personal neatness, psychosocial and mental function, and depression.

The results indicate a dramatic difference between the two groups. The residents who interacted with the puppies improved in six out of eight areas measured. Francis and Turner were not surprised by their findings and noted further that it is fairly well documented that animals are therapeutically effective with various populations and in various settings. The affected, measured variables could be said to be indications of quality of life. If one accepts this, the study has shown that a simplistic, inexpensive, "treatment" modality can significantly improve psychosocial function, hence, "quality of life" (Odean and Cussack, p. 14).

These 3 studies were of particular interest to the authors as the introduction of pets to the elderly in a variety of settings has the potential of improving the quality of life of participants in the day care setting and secondly, this therapeutic modality is inexpensive. The expense of any modality is a prime concern for program planning in an adult day care center.

The first introduction of an animal to the program came from a visit of a poodle owned by the program receptionist in 1982. This highly active, gentle animal piqued the interest of the majority of participants, but because of this dog's high energy level, the dog was not suitable for this very sedentary population. Clearly, the general response to this animal was strong and positive, stimulating much discussion and more interest than previously observed following other special events. During the period in which the concept of starting a visitation program was discussed with the day care staff, the inevitable objections arose. Each potential problem and question had to be addressed and given merit before proceeding toward implementation.

One staff member felt it might be "illegal" to have a dog at any adult daycare in the state of North Carolina. It is not stated in the North Carolina Adult Daycare Certification Regulations that animals are prohibited on the premises of adult day care centers. Nor are there any policies from the umbrella organization, the Coordinating Council for Senior Citizens, that disallowed animals on the program site. The church in which the program is housed, Duke Memorial Methodist, saw no objection.

Another fear voiced by staff was that participants of low intelligence or with dementing illnesses would be afraid of a dog. (In fact, it was the particular staff members' own fears that had brought this problem to the surface.) Curiosity replaced fear for the staff, and this was reflected by the retarded as well as the more normal participants. The authors felt it was most important to elicit information from staff members as well as participants as to their past interactions with pets since the effects of negative attitudes of both the participant and staff members could influence the total group.

With these initial concerns settled, the coordinator arranged for the Durham Kennel Club to stage a mini-performance of obedience of their animals for the participants at the day care program. This was an ideal way to introduce reluctant staff members and participants to the inclusions of animals at the facility.

The "Durham Kennel Club Super Dog" show was received enthusiastically by staff and participants. Five dogs were accompanied by four masters. One dog, a beautiful English spaniel, was a famous dog who had appeared in dog food television commercials and on the label of Milkbone Dog biscuit box. This dog was thirteen years old and had developed difficulty in seeing and hearing. Touchingly, the participants of this program for the elderly identified with the dog's condition and were very forgiving of his mistake during his performance.

Two very affectionate Highland terriers were a highlight. One participant, Ms. L., was very attracted to these dogs and approached the owner of the dog to help her with the performance. Ms. L. was awarded the duty of holding one dog while the other was put through its paces. She was visibly proud and spoke out to others whenever she could make eye contact.

Two large dogs, a German shepherd and a young boxer, were also part of the program. The gentlemen, Mr. G., Mr. E., Mr. J., and Mr. S., were interested and petted the dogs as soon as they came within reach. Mr. E. was very verbal at this point and told about his own dog, Wolf, and regaled the group with tales of Wolf's prowess and viciousness.

During the actual demonstration, each of the 26 participants and 6 staff members present were respectful, quiet, interested and remarkably alert.

This introduction served more than one function. First, it introduced animals to the participants in a controlled fashion. Dog and master were a team and each was disciplined and experienced. Second, it allowed staff's anxiety to be recognized. And third, it gave time to both staff and participants to direct questions about dogs and their care and training to experts. One participant asked "How come little dogs are so wound up (excitable)?" Another asked "When is it too late to train a dog?" One staff member asked, "What diseases can you get from a dog?" All questions, though sometimes amusing to the Kennel Club members, were answered thoroughly and respectfully. This was an extremely good way to "set the stage" for animal visitation.

TAME WILD ANIMALS

Shortly after the Kennel Club's program, a special tame "wild" animal show was arranged through the Durham Museum of Life and Science. Because the participants had so thoroughly enjoyed their other experience with animals, they looked forward to meeting and "greeting" the wild animals.

On the scheduled day, all but one of the participants were present in the Day room. Most were anxiously awaiting the appearance of the first animal. The first wild animal to be introduced was a CHICKEN. There was much joking among the participants, who were generally fascinated with the chicken. Most would touch the chicken and cooperate with the handler. The chicken was a big hit especially with Virgie, a farmer's wife and Ella (now blind) who was reared on a farm.

The rabbit was the next animal introduced. Most participants touched the rabbit but the rabbit was most appealing to the blind participants who would constantly stroke the rabbit's fur and comment on its softness. Observers noted that there was little reminiscence or conversation.

When the third animal, the opposum, was introduced there was hesitation to touch it until the coordinator initiated the action. Then all of the participants seemed to want to pet the opposum. Eva, a participant, took the opposum onto her own lap while another participant recalled many past opposum meals. Many of the women remembered cooking opposum during "hard" times. None of the participants remembered "tame" opposums. The conversation level during this period was very high, with many conversations at one time. Not one of the participants fell asleep during the afternoon.

An announcement was made that the last wild animal was to be a 5 foot King snake. Three of the participants left the room. All of the remaining 27 appeared very interested. Silent staring was followed by vigorous conversation, laughing and startled responses. Eva petted the snake, took it from the handler and placed it upon her head. Many of the participants lost much of their fear and reminisced about snakes in "corn cribs" and barns that were beneficial. This was a very stimulating and bonding experience. The general feeling was one of shared awe and fascination. One participant expressed anxiety but remained. Another participant stood in the doorway for the duration of the program, and laughed and watched every moment. This experience remained in the memory of most of the participants the following day.

The authors noted many positive outcomes from the two animals programs: greater participation during the program, increased attention span, and increased memory of the program a day later. Also staff appeared to be responding and interacting with the participants more positively than previously noted. With such positive results, the impossibility of establishing a regular visitation schedule at this time with the Kennel Club due to lack of available volunteers was very disheartening. Despite this setback, we decided to establish a temporary program that would help keep the interests of the participants high.

We selected another privately owned pet, Bridget, a three year old Irish setter. Having been abused and abandoned at six months, Bridget remained with the town veterinarian for another 6 months until a suitable home was found. After 2 years in a children-filled household, Bridget was a loving docile animal. She spent most of her day looking for someone to stroke her fur or scratch her ears and belly. She was considered to be a most appropriate pet for visitation.

TARGETED INDIVIDUALS WITH BRIDGET

Those participants who had been exhibiting isolating and withdrawn behavior seemed the subjects who might be best observed directly with the animal. Three participants over 78 years old were initially chosen by the day care coordinator as individuals showing these behaviors; they also had owned animals, dogs and cats, and remembered the animals fondly when questioned. Only one of these 3 participants currently lived with a dog in her home, cared for by her grandchildren. All of these participants manifesting withdrawal and isolation had been diagnosed as suffering from Alzheimer's disease. They were assigned a very simple task: they were asked to hold the dog's leash for fifteen minutes. The individuals were spaced in 3 different sections of the general meeting room. Those other staff and participants interested in the individual and/or dog were able to come and go at their leisure. The facilitator and investigator observed the interactions and recorded them. But at all times a sense of "naturalness" was of the utmost concern.

On the first visit, when Bridget entered with the handler through the vestibule, few participants were aware of their entrance. Spending ten minutes in the reception area allowed the news of their arrival to travel through the group. An introduction of Bridget to the participants in the general meeting room was done only once at the initial visit. (This gentle, attractive, and friendly animal was a favorite at once with a large number of non-targeted individuals.) After the introduction the animal was directed to Mr. S. The investigator pressed the leash into the hand and a warm smile showed the appreciation of being allowed to be with Bridget. Each of those given the dog seemed to accept the responsibility positively. The greatest difficulty encountered was that those not

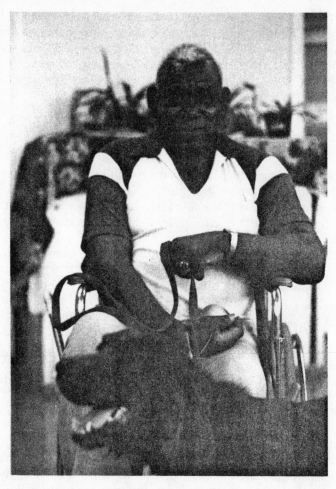

For those individuals regularly invited to hold Bridget, the experience became a source of pride and personal reward.

targeted wanted to hold the dog and sometimes tried to take his leash.

R.S.

This gentleman of 83 had been a very active member of the community as a younger man; however, the progress of Alzheimer's disease had left him isolated and withdrawn. Because of his attractive disposition and numerous intact social skills, R.S. had been maintained in the day care program. Despite increasing loss of cognitive ability, R.S. had enjoyed a secure retirement; having worked as a supervisor in the local tobacco company for many years, he earned a substantial pension. A homeowner with a monthly income over $500, this widower was one of the most prosperous of the program participants, although this might not be evident from his appearance. Living alone made him a victim of thieves and vandals; sadly it had been determined that thieves were invited into the home by R.S. himself. Most recently R.S. had suffered from an aggravated hernia condition. Although surgery had been scheduled, the hernia had been unlocatable to physicians not a week before the pet visitation program was to begin.

Observations of Bridget's visits and the participants response to her are noted here. R.S. began reminiscing while petting Bridget. These reminisces were concerned with his having trained hunting dogs in the past; family members and the pets they had owned; he talked considerably about a special dog he had given his daughter. R. S. was also very verbal during his time with Bridget. He reported about an episode of pain over the weekend which required hospitalization. The coordinator especially noted this as R.S. had never reported any information to the program until this time. Throughout the morning Mr. S. maintained more interest in conversations with other participants. When asked if he recalled the visitors of the morning an hour after their departure, he recalled only that a dog had come to the program. He did not recall the name of the dog nor that a handler had accompanied the dog. Mr. S. remained wakeful throughout the afternoon and still recalled the visitation of the dog at the close of the program that day at 3:30 P.M. The following day, Mr. S. was asked if he remembered anything special from the day before and his response was a smiling "Oh yes, oh yes." He did not appear to remember the dog visit, but rather something pleasant had occurred.

J.U.

Another Alzheimer's victim, this black woman was unable to communicate except in sentence fragments. The fragments almost never were comprehensible, partly because she stam-

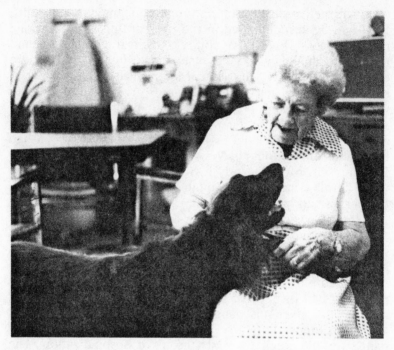

No one was exempt from Bridget's charm. The dog appealed to the participants regardless of handicap.

mered in a heavy Southern dialect, but primarily because she did not seem able to find words for her thoughts. She was very isolated by her disorder, although she did not appear to be in distress. She had few interactions with other participants or staff. A month before the pet visitation program was to begin, a blind participant to whom Mrs. U. had been very attached was placed in a nursing home. Although both women suffered from dementing disorders, they had found comfort and companionship with one another through touch and care. After her companion's removal from the program, Mrs. U.'s isolation became more evident, although the manifestations of her illness had not changed. In appearance, Mrs. U. was eccentric, always wearing a turban-like head gear and a handmade apron. Once or twice a week, she would be seen rocking, swaying alone, and seemingly singing religious music. Although the activity was not focused on the activities transpiring in the larger group, her behavior was accepted as normal by other elderly participants, but the staff generally found this activity disconcerting. Mrs. U. was not stimulated to conversation, but seemed to exhibit focused smiling behavior toward the dog Bridget and her handler during the visiting sessions. She expressed her interest in the animal by walking with the dog in the meeting room and the corridor. Mrs. U. smiled at staff and participants during the hour following the visit and sat for lunch with the most active of the group members. When asked if she remembered the visit of the dog, she was able to remember it one hour after the dog had left but was unable to remember the animal by the afternoon. The following day, Mrs. U. did not respond to the question concerning the visit the day before. Mrs. U. repeated her seating with the active group and smiled and nodded to others throughout the day.

J.L.

This woman had been a active member of the group one year before but had increasingly withdrawn into reading activities. When asked what she had read she could seldom recall even the name of the book or magazine. Adding to her withdrawal and memory loss due to Alzheimer's disease was a severe hearing loss. Wearing a hearing aid did not alleviate the handicap since the device was always turned off or in some way did not function. A family situation had made it impossible for Mrs. L. to remain in her home and this woman had finally found a reliable caregiving relative in her niece. She had lived with this niece and the niece's grandchildren since her enrollment at the daycare center. This element of dislocation and alien environment has been clear to the staff and her family. A dog in her home was often her companion. At the daycare program, she had not developed any attachments to individuals or staff members that could be described as substantive or close. The presence of the dog in the facility was arousing to Mrs. L. When the dog arrived at the program, Mrs. L. became more animated and showed a distinct mood change. She conversed with participants and staff about the dog. She asked to hold the dog, and she attempted to instruct those chosen to hold the dog on the proper handling

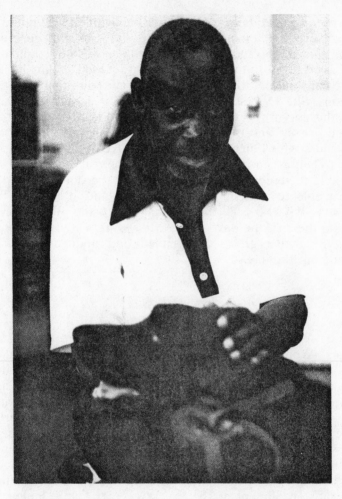

Stroking the coat of this attractive, well-groomed animal was enticing to the individuals in the program.

of the animal. When she was allowed to hold the dog's leash, she was most animated and her conversations with others were about the dog Bridget in present time. When asked if she had a dog in her own home, she could not recall it. One hour after the visit, she clearly recalled and recounted the dog in detailed physical description. Her elevated mood remained throughout the day and extended to the pantomime activities of the afternoon. By afternoon, she could not remember the visit of the morning. The following day she did not recall the animal had visited.

For Mrs. L., each visit elicited the elevated change in mood. Although she was not able to recall the actual visit, she did seem to be familiar with the dog on succeeding visits. During the period the dog was in the program, Mrs. L. conversed about the dog to others as a recognized object. She knew the dog when she saw it, and recounted the dog's past behavior when the dog was present.

CONCLUSION

This study revealed findings similar to those conducted by Robb and Francis, that pets can be catalysts for social behavior. These clients with Alzheimer's disease were withdrawn,

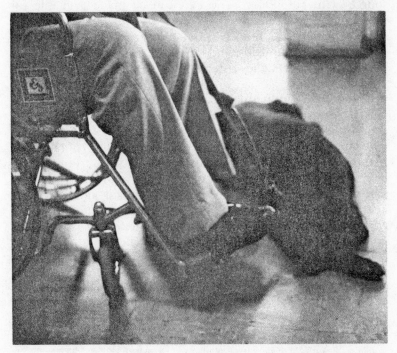

Mutual trust and non-verbal communication which developed, as well as the generous, non-judgmental affection of this dog made her a welcome visitor to the day program.

self-centered and uncommunicative. These clients had not responded to previous therapeutic methods. Yet after the various pet programs as well as visits with Bridget, observations were made in the areas of increased verbalization, smiling, attention to pet, increased periods of "awakeness" after pet left the site.

Mary Opal Wolanin made the observation that virtually all the interactional therapies (group, music, poetry, recreational therapy, etc.) adapted from psychiatric settings to the care of older, confused, withdrawn clients have been effective. She believes that success relates to the feeling of personhood or being a part of the human community that results. These therapies work, not by doing anything to the person, but rather by removing the barriers that keep people from being free to be themselves in the environment.

The use of pets for therapeutic purposes represents an interactional therapy that draws upon an abundant resource. Unwanted dogs and cats can be made available for more hours at a much lower cost and in greater numbers than psychiatrists, nurses, poets, and others, the cost of veterinary care, housing and training not withstanding. Thus pet therapy meets the criterion for sustainability (Wolanin, 1982).

Today many individuals lack human companionship. Some lack purpose and productivity. A simple addition of a pet who eagerly awaits one and responds to one's care and attention may mean the difference between maintaining contact with reality and withdrawal (Searles, 1960). Pets are effective in increasing patient responsiveness, giving patients a pleasurable experience, enhancing treatment milieu and they help keep patients in touch with reality (Levinson, 1969). As a result, staff efforts are rendered more successful and gratifying and rapport with patients and staff could be aided with the use of animals.

REFERENCES

Andrysco, Robert M., "Pet Facilitative Therapy in a Retirement Nursing Community," Presentation at 1981 International Conference on Human/Companion Animal Bond, October 5–7, 1981, Philadelphia, PA.

Cussack, Odean and Smith, Elaine, Pets and the Elderly—The Therapeutic Bond, Activities, Adaptation and Aging, Vol. 4, No. 2/3, January, 1984, Haworth Press.

Francis, Gloria; Turner, Jean T.; Johnson, Suzanne B.; "Domestic Animals Visitation as Therapy with Adult Home Residents," unpublished report.

Robb, Suzanne; Boyd, Michele; Pristash, Carole Lee; "A Wine Bottle, Plant and Puppy: Catalysts for Social Behavior," Journal of Gerontological Nursing, 6 (12), December, 1980.

Living With Dying:
A Model for Helping
Nursing Home Residents and Staff
Deal With Death

Adele Weiner

ABSTRACT. This paper presents a two component, inter-disciplinary model for helping nursing home residents deal with their own impending deaths and that of their friends and relatives. The first step involves an active, overt funeral and burial planning process and the second step involves the actual funeral. This is described in detail so that it can be applied in a variety of other residential settings.

Nursing Homes have long been characterized as being "places to die" and it is true that for many individuals, the nursing home is their final residence. However, for some residents, the long term care facility serves as their home for an extended period of time. During this period, they develop meaningful relationships with other people. Yet, they are residing in a setting where it is likely that many of the friends they make will die. Thus, not only must these nursing home residents plan for their own deaths and resolve the psychosocial task of "Integrity vs. Despair,"[1] but they also may have to deal with a series of deaths of significant others.

This article presents a model of inter-disciplinary professional practice designed to help the residents, and indirectly

Adele Weiner, ACSW, Assistant Professor of Social Work, is a member of the faculty of the Westchester Social Work Education Consortium and the former Chairperson of the Social Work Department, King's College, Wilkes-Barre, Pennsylvania. She is the former Director of Social Services at the Brooklyn United Methodist Church Home, Brooklyn, New York, where this model was developed. Please address inquiries to: P.O. Box 1186, Old Chelsea Station, New York, NY 10113.

the staff, deal with the multiple deaths that occur in nursing homes. It is proposed that this model is not unique to the particular home in which it was used and developed but rather is applicable within all long term care facilities. It works best with patients who are fairly alert and it can be modified according to the professional's assessment of the patient's coping abilities and emotional state. It can be implemented without increasing the work loads of staff or requiring additional funds.

Underlying this model is the assumption that by helping residents resolve issues about death, their lives in the nursing home will be more meaningful. This incorporates a wholistic philosophy that recognizes that in addition to meeting the biological/medical needs of residents, it is also necessary to focus concern on the psychosocial/emotional and spiritual/religious needs of residents. Such a view of care helps to prevent the "social death" that often occurs in institutional settings long before the actual biological death.

Often the application process or actual admission to a long term care facility symbolically begins the process of dying that Kubler-Ross has identified.[2] For these individuals, the need for institutional placement, or the actuality of that placement, confronts the individual with the reality of mortality. Residents can go through the stages of denial, anger, bargaining, depression and acceptance[3] in response to this symbolic indication of impending death.

Complicating the individual's resolution of these tasks is the process of institutionalization or depersonalization, which is inherent in the structure of institutional living.[4] The individual entering the nursing home has suffered multiple losses prior to admission to the facility, and once in the home, will experience continuing multiple losses due to their declining health and the deaths of friends and relatives.

This model presupposes that the individual will benefit from support and the opportunity to discuss their losses and plan for his/her own death. This model has two major components: (1) funeral/burial planning and (2) the funeral/memorial service itself.

The process begins when the social worker, or other designated individual, meets with individuals to complete a "Burial Arrangement Form," which is probably already in use in some facilities. Using the form as a tool, the worker can open up discussion of the individual's planning for death.[5] While the information that such forms provide is useful and necessary, these facts are usually secondary to the utilization of the form as an opening to allow residents to discuss death. In the hands of a sensitive worker, such a task-oriented approach can provide the resident with a powerful psychosocial experience without incorporating the threatening stigma of "counseling or therapy."

Residents seem to be relieved that someone is concerned about their final requests and plans. Those without families are often worried and concerned about whether their plans will be carried out. Those with families are usually concerned about the expense to their family and want to make plans that will ease the situation when the time comes. Sometimes, there is a concern about conflict within the family and the residents are pleased to have the opportunity to have their wishes known. At this time, residents also have the opportunity, with the help of the staff, to make arrangements for funerals and burials or other services. Financial arrangements can also be made to prepay for funerals, cemetary plots or monuments.

For those residents who have no relatives, or designated person, the administrator of the home, the business manager and/or social worker make the final arrangements when necessary. This assures the resident that they will be taken care of according to their wishes.

When a resident with family dies, the family is informed of the wishes of the resident. Often they are already aware of the arrangements and have the necessary forms and documents. But sometimes, if they have not yet planned or if they had little recent contact with the deceased, they are grateful to have a copy of the burial arrangements form with the resident's plans and wishes. (See Table 1.) It may also inform them of important information such as the location of the cemetery plots and/or the location of the deed, and arrangements made with monument makers or funeral directors. These forms serve the purpose of easing the resident's mind and assisting the family in an organized way with practical, necessary information at a time of trauma.

The usefulness of this form is not solely with the information it provides. The social worker can use it as a means of

TABLE 1

SAMPLE BURIAL ARRANGEMENTS FORM

THIS FORM HAS BEEN DEVELOPED TO LET YOU INFORM US OF ANY PLANS YOU
HAVE ALREADY MADE OR WISH TO MAKE CONCERNING YOUR FUNERAL AND BURIAL.
THE STAFF IS AVAILABLE TO HELP YOU MAKE ARRANGEMENTS. PLEASE ANSWER
ALL THE QUESTIONS THAT APPLY:

NAME _____

WHO SHOULD WE CONTACT TO TAKE CARE OF YOUR FUNERAL AND BURIAL?:
      NAME _____
      ADDRESS _____
      TELEPHONE _____
      RELATIONSHIP TO YOU _____

IS THERE A CHURCH OR CLERGY MEMBER THAT SHOULD BE NOTIFIED?
      NAME _____
      ADDRESS _____
      TELEPHONE _____

DO YOU HAVE A CEMETARY PLOT?
IF YES: LOCATION OF CEMETARY PLOT?_____
      DEED NUMBER?_____
      WHERE IS DEED?_____
      WHAT FINANCIAL ARRANGEMENTS HAVE BEEN OR NEED TO BE
      MADE?_____

HAVE YOU MAD ANY PLANS FOR A MONUMENT?
IF YES: NAME OF MONUMENT MAKER _____
      ADDRESS _____
      TELEPHONE _____
      WHAT FINANCIAL ARRANGEMENTS HAVE BEEN OR NEED TO BE
      MADE?_____

WHAT FUNERAL HOME DO YOU WISH TO BE USED?
      NAME OF FUNERAL HOME _____
      ADDRESS _____
      TELEPHONE _____
      WHAT FINANCIAL ARRANGEMENTS HAVE BEEN OR NEED TO BE
      MADE? _____

DO YOU BELONG TO A BURIAL SOCIETY?
IF YES: WHO IS TO BE CONTACTED? _____
      ADDRESS _____
      TELEPHONE _____
      ARE THERE ANY FURTHER ARRANGEMENTS THAT NEED
      TO BE MADE? _____

DO YOU HAVE A LIFE INSURANCE POLICY OR HAVE MADE OTHER FINANCIAL
ARRANGEMENTS TO PAY FOR YOUR FUNERAL/BURIAL?
      INSURANCE COMPANY _____
      ADDRESS _____
      TELEPHONE _____
      POLICY NUMBER _____
      LOCATION OF POLICY _____

TABLE 1, continued

```
ANY OTHER FINANCIAL PLANS MADE FOR FUNERAL/BURIAL (VA
BENEFITS, PREPAID PLAN, ETC.):




HAVE YOU MADE ANY PLANS OR WISH TO MAKE ANY PLANS TO BE CREMATED
OR TO DONATE YOUR BODY OR BODY PARTS. PLEASE DESCRIBE ANY WISHES
OR PLANS:
    HAVE THE NECESSARY FORMS OR DOCUMENTS BEEN SIGNED?




PLEASE DESCIRBE ANY PLANS YOU HAVE FOR YOUR FUNERAL OR BURIAL,
SUCH AS LOCATION OF SERVICES, SPECIAL MUSIC, FLOWERS, ITEMS YOU
WISH BURIED WITH YOU, ETC.




I HAVE READ THE ABOVE INFORMATION CONCERNING MY PLANS AND WISHES FOR
MY BURIAL/FUNERAL. IF MY RELATIVES ARE UNABLE TO CARRY OUT MY
PLANS/WISHES, I AUTHORIZE THE ADMINISTRATOR OF THE HOME TO PROCEED
WITH MY FUNERAL/BURIAL AS DESCRIBED ABOVE.
                              SIGNED _____
WITNESS _____  DATE _____
```

affording the resident the opportunity to talk about their anxieties and concerns about death. Often, they discuss spouses, whom they have lost or are concerned with, and their plans to be together.

Mrs. C was a 70 year old Hispanic woman, who was alert and aware. She was a very proud woman and had always taken care of herself and her husband, when he was alive. She had decided to enter the nursing home after her husband's death. When the worker went to discuss her burial arrangements, Mrs. C produced a bill from the monument maker, indicating that the monument for her husband was completed and installed. She was concerned about making sure that it was correct, but she had no family to take care of this for her. So the social worker and Mrs. C went to the cemetery to visit her husband. Afterwards, both went to the monument maker to pay the bill and make sure that all the arrangements were made for her headstone. Throughout this activity she talked about her husband and their life together and seemed comforted and eased in knowing that everything was planned.

As this example presents, it is fairly easy to incorporate the pragmatic, practical aspects of funeral planning with a concern to the emotional/spiritual needs of the resident. Once the resident has had the opportunity to make plans and discuss other concerns about death, they need not expend excessive psychic energy on these issues and can continue on with the work of living.

The second major component of this model concerns the actual funerals or other services for the residents. The funeral, as a social ritual, offers friends and family the opportunity to say goodbye and serves a valuable function in the grieving process.[5] In nursing homes, where residents are debilitated, they are often deprived of the opportunity to say goodbye to their friends and the social support of funeral/burial rituals. If there are no relatives, the friends in the nursing home, and the staff, may be the only ones who may mourn the death of an individual.

The home in which this model was used had a small chapel, and whenever possible, we encouraged the family to use it for the funeral or a memorial service. In cases where there was no family, the funeral was always held in the chapel, unless the resident had made specific other plans. In situations where family preferred to have the funeral at another location, the residents held their own memorial service in the chapel. The staff also participated.

Such memorial services, and many of the funeral services, were planned and organized by a group of residents who had also taken the responsibility for the weekly, inter-denominational prayer meetings. Friends and family members of the deceased were also included in this planning process. The residents and family members were assisted in this task by the appropriate clergy and the recreation, nursing and social services staff. The format of these services included eulogies, poetry readings, the singing of songs and hymns and appropriate religious functions. This type of service would be possible in facilities without chapels and would offer the residents the opportunity to say their goodbyes. The residents are encouraged and assisted to take an active role in this entire process in order to support their emotional and spiritual needs.

Another important aspect of the actual funeral activities is to let the living residents know that they will also be cared for and missed. As part of the planning process, the resident had the opportunity to designate which suit/dress they would like to be buried in, songs they would like sung, flowers, etc. It is important for the living residents to see that these wishes are carried out. The social worker or other staff member, in some cases family, and the residents who were friends of the deceased, picked out appropriate clothing for the burial and other things of importance to the deceased (jewelry, rosaries, Bibles, etc). The Head of Housekeeping would get the designated suit/dress and ensure that it was cleaned and given to the Funeral Director.

If the funeral was to be in the home and the coffin was open, prior to the service the social worker or other staff member would go with residents to view the person in the chapel. This was to see how the deceased looked and how well the Funeral Director had done his/her job. This is extremely important because the residents learn that others will make sure that everything is just right for them. It also gives them the opportunity to do one final thing for the deceased.

> Mrs. D had been a loud, often disruptive resident, who was not liked by some residents. Her death had been due to her denial of medical treatment and her harrassment of the staff, which had been witnessed by many other residents. She had been a chain smoker, and when it came time to select her burial dress, it was difficult to find a nice dress without burn holes. When the residents went to see how she looked for her funeral, one noticed a burn hole right in the front of her dress. Without saying anything, another resident went over to the vase of flowers, took out a rose and placed it across Mrs. D so

that the burn was covered. The resident then placed
Mrs. D's rosary in the coffin with the flower.

Finally, the residents were active in participating in the
actual service. They played the piano, sang hymns, interacted
with family and made short speeches on behalf of the deceased. Most families felt that the participation of the nursing
homes residents, who had interacted on a daily basis with the
deceased, added a dimension of "humaness" to the service
and were glad to know of the meaning of their relatives' lives
to others.

Alternatives exist for those homes that do not have chapels, for it is important for the residents to have the opportunity to say "goodbye" to their friends in a supportive environment. Memorial meetings can be held in a day room or
the recreation room, using clergy, social work and recreation
staff. Such services are appropriate for severely debilitated
residents who could not attend a funeral outside of the nursing home. It is important to allow the residents, even those
who are often considered "senile," the opportunity to have
the social supports incorporated into such services. Very
often disoriented residents function appropriately and ade-
quately within the structure of formalized religious/social
rituals, which serve as a form of reality orientation. Of
course, special efforts should be made to support the psychosocial functioning of those residents who may have limited
emotional/spiritual resources to depend on. Yet it is these
same residents who have reduced psychosocial functioning,
who need the most support from the staff to deal with their
grief and are usually ignored in funerals, since it is often
assumed that "they don't know what is happening."

It is also important for the staff to know the role the decreased served in the life of the living residents. For example,
if the deceased was an alert resident that helped others in
activities or at meals it may be necessary for the staff to
replace these functions, using either staff, volunteers, family
or other residents. This is necessary in order to prevent further deterioration of the living residents that would be pre-
cipitated by factors that complicate the grieving process.

If the funeral home is located near the nursing home and
residents can be transported to the services, they should be

offered the opportunity to attend. Nursing home staff may have to intervene with family members, who may have feelings about residents attending.

In conclusion, this model has as an underlying premise the naturalness of death and its place in the life cycle. Death is "the final stage of growth"[6] and dealing with it allows individuals to continue living. Social rituals have been developed that meet the emotional and spiritual needs of individuals faced with death, and in institutional settings in which the residents are both debilitated and faced with death on a continuous basis, staff need to work together to support the residents in the resolution of tasks related to their own and others' deaths. Focused around two major sets of activities—funeral planning and actual services—this inter-disciplinary approach strives to meet the medical/biological, psychosocial/emotional and religious/spiritual needs of the residents in order to maximize their continuing growth and development.

REFERENCES

1. Erik H. Erikson, *Identity, Youth and Crisis*, New York: W.W. Norton & Company, 1968, pp. 139–141.
2. Elizabeth Kubler-Ross, *On Death and Dying*, New York: MacMillan Publishing Company, 1969.
3. Ibid.
4. Marcella B. Weiner, Albert J. Brok, and Alvin M. Snadowsky, *Working With the Aged: Practical Approaches in the Institution and Community*, Englewood Cliffs, New Jersey: Prentice Hall, 1978.
5. James E. Eddy and Wesley F. Alles, *Death Education*, St. Louis, Missouri: C.V. Mosby Company, 1983, and Kathy Charmaz, *The Social Realities of Death: Death in Contemporary America*, Reading, Massachusetts: Addison-Wesley Publishing, 1980, pp. 199–204.
6. Elizabeth Kubler-Ross, *Death: The Final Stage of Growth*, Englewood Cliffs, New Jersey: Prentice Hall, 1975.

The Relationship Between Nursing Home Residents' Perceptions of Nursing Staff and Quality of Nursing Home Care

Shayna Stein
Margaret W. Linn
Elliott M. Stein

ABSTRACT. The purpose of the study was to determine if nursing home patients' perception of nursing staff members were associated with quality of nursing home care. Three hospital professional staff members who were familiar with the homes in the study rated the 10 homes on a 1 = excellent to 4 = poor quality. Patients (N = 239) admitted to the 10 homes provided assessments after they had been in the nursing home for one month of the nursing staff activities. Homes were classified by the four levels of care and responses of the patients were compared by multivariate analysis of variance. Patient responses differed significantly among the four levels of quality, with significantly more favorable responses in the excellent homes and the least favorable in the poor homes. In poorer homes, patients perceived less respect, communication, response from calls, concern, and also believed staff members did not like their work. In addition, when asked how the staff would respond to specific situations, patients in poorer quality homes less often selected the more favorable behaviors. The study demonstrates that patients are able to assess quality by

Dr. Shayna Stein is Social Science Researcher, Veterans Administration Medical Center, and Adjunct Instructor with the Department of Psychiatry, University of Miami School of Medicine, Miami, FL. Dr. Linn is Director, Social Science Research, Veterans Administration Medical Center, and Professor of Psychiatry at the University of Miami School of Medicine. Dr. Elliot Stein is Director of Psychiatric Services of The Douglas Gardens Community Mental Health Center of Miami Beach, and Clinical Assistant Professor with the Department of Psychiatry, University of Miami School of Medicine.

This project was funded by Veterans Administration Health Services Research and Development Grant No. 547.

their perceptions of nursing staff and suggests that patients' assessments should be included in evaluations of homes. Further, it points up the need for in-service training in attempting to enhance the quality of care.

Nursing homes represent one of the most exciting frontiers for change in medical and nursing care today. No one can realistically doubt that the increased need for nursing home beds and the economic constraints of our society will combine to require creative and intelligent planning if future health care delivery for the infirm elderly is to be responsive and humane. Already change is evident. Over the last 15 years, the importance of assessing the quality of nursing home care has gained added attention[1-3] with some research linked to specific interventions and their outcomes.[4] Studies concerning nursing home utilization,[5,6] manpower needs,[7] effects of innovative programming,[8] family involvement in care,[9,10] and patient outcomes over time[11] have been among those contributing information of potential benefit to nursing home patients.

Most of the literature evaluating nursing home care has focused on patient adjustment by examining a variety of physical and psychological factors. There has been little attention paid to the residents' own perceptions of the nursing home environment. One notable exception to this is a study of stress, coping, and survival by Lieberman and Tobin.[12] Results showed that environmental factors were crucial to the well being of a less "docile" subgroup of institutionalized patients. These factors included warmth and recognition. Patients showing less "aged" behavioral patterns were most responsive to environmental qualities. In another study by Simms et al.,[13] outcomes showed that the residents' perceptions of the nursing home influenced their subsequent adjustment.

Quality of extended, long-term, or nursing home care has received relatively little research attention compared with hospital care. Nursing home studies vary by their definitions of quality. Early studies measured quality by observation,[14] social climate,[15] physician hours,[16] panels of judges using specific weighted criteria,[17] interactions between staff and patients,[18] and available resources in the home.[19] The bricks-and-mortar-type variables were considered a "structural" type of evaluation and used alone were generally an unsatisfactory indicator of quality, given the fact that certain minimal structural elements were met. At the other end of the quality of care measurement continuum was "patient outcome" types of evaluation. Studies of outcomes of nursing home patients,[20,21] however, were long-term and expensive, with outcomes including such factors for assessment as death, disease, disability, discomfort, and dissatisfaction, referred to by White[22] as the five D's of evaluation. Between the structural and outcome types of evaluation fall "process" methods. Process type of assessment assumes that persons responsible for organizing care can agree on what constitutes high quality without actual measuring outcome. As might be expected, process evaluation has recieved considerable attention, including such methods as quality audits through peer review, utilization studies, cost studies, or direct observations.

Process evaluation has been done by both implicit and explicit methods. *Implicit* judgments are usually global assessments of care provided from records or by observation. *Explicit* methods involve experts setting detailed criteria for quality of care related to specific diagnoses or types of care. In 1974, one of us studied[23] the relationship between implicit global judgements of six social workers about 40 nursing homes and explicit ratings obtained on structural and process variables recorded on a 71-item Nursing Home Rating Scale.[24] Using stepwise regression techniques, implicit ratings were predicted significantly from the explicit subscores that described the physical plant, dietary practices, administrative policies, and staff-patient ratios. Agreement between the six social workers' implicit ratings was a Kendall W of .85. Thus, there was considerable agreement among the raters as well as between the methods of assessment. In a study of outcomes of 1,000 patients[20] placed in nursing homes, professional nursing hours per patient, dietary practices, and staff-patient ratios were associated with better patient outcomes. Therefore, the predictors of implicit ratings by explicit criteria were similar to those that were found to be related to patient outcome.

In the present study, quality was defined by implicit ratings made for a group of nursing homes by an external team. Nursing home residents' perceptions of the nursing staff and specific behaviors of staff were collected in these homes. The purpose of the study was to determine whether the patients' evaluations were associated significantly with the external evaluations of quality of care provided for the homes.

METHOD

Data collection took place over a three-year period in 10 community skilled nursing homes selected to provide variations in number of beds, staff members, and admissions per month. Homes were in Miami, Florida, and were visited by a research nurse who screened all patients admitted to the homes. Those who were not expected to remain for an extended time and those who were too sick to respond were excluded. Demographic information concerning age, sex, race, education, marital status, and income were collected. After the patients had been in the home for one month, they completed two scales evaluating nursing staff in the home. The first scale contained six items that concerned nursing staff responsiveness: treated with respect; likes their work; someone from staff that is special to the patient; how soon staff respond when called; staff liking you; and someone from staff with whom the person could talk. Patients rated each item from 1 to 5, with a higher score representing a less favorable rating. Principal component factor analysis of this scale showed all items loaded heavily (from .51 to .78) on one factor, allowing for the use of a total score or indicating high correlations among the variables. Thus, a general patient response to nursing staff was reflected by the ratings.

The second instrument asked for the patients to indicate what they thought the nurses in their homes would do if faced with three specific situations. Patients were asked to place a mark by the response which best represented what they believed the majority of nurses would do in *their home* if confronted by these situations: (1) if patient is feeling angry and expresses anger to the nurse, the nurse would probably (leave the room and give the patient time to calm down, point out all the things the patient has to be grateful for, or mention the anger and ask if they can help*); (2) sometimes sick people feel that they are being punished by God, and the patient says that this is the way he or she feels, the nurse would probably (mention God works in mysterious ways and no one can know his will, encourage the patient to talk about his or her feelings,* or tell patient not to talk that way because it will only make the feelings worse); and (3) the patient wants to know more about his physical condition and so asks the nurse, the nurse would probably (leave that up to the doctor, tell the patient not to dwell on the illness, or approach the patient and find out how ill he is feeling*). The asterisk after the response indicates the one selected as most often being the correct response. Thus, each of the three variables were scored 0 for incorrect and 1 for a correct response.

Two individuals were selected to independently rate the overall quality of care provided by the 10 homes in the study. A nurse who visited these and other community nursing homes regularly as a member of an inspection team was selected. In addition, two social workers who provided followup services to patients in nursing homes after placement from the hospital were chosen. The social workers had been seeing patients in the homes for about 10 years. All were staff members of the Veterans Administration Medical Center in Miami and were not involved in the present study in any other way. They were asked to rate the 10 homes in the study independently from 1 = excellent to 4 = poor overall quality. They were instructed to use their knowledge about all aspects of the home and care provided as a basis for the ratings. Agreement between one of the social workers and the nurse was high (r = .80 by intraclass correlation). Homes were grouped by quality ratings into four categories for analysis, with the other social worker's rating serving as the deciding category for those homes in which there was not perfect agreement. Two homes were classified as excellent, four as good, two as fair, and two as poor quality. It should be mentioned that the homes in the sample probably could be considered as providing a broad range of care with none actually being the very worst in the nursing home industry or perhaps the very best.

Data were analysed in the following ways: (1) Patient characteristics were correlated (Pearson r's) with responses to both patient scales. In addition, patient characteristics were compared between the four classifications of quality of care. That is, patients in excellent quality homes were compared with those in the good, fair, and poor homes. If significant relationships were found, covariance would have been used in further analyses comparing the quality of care groups (use of covariance adjusts for confounding effects of other variables correlated with the dependent variable[25]). (2) Using multivariate analysis of variance, the patient responses in the four classifications of quality of care homes were compared to determine if patient responses differentiated significantly in the expected directions among the four groups.

RESULTS

Description of Patients and Relationship of Patient Characteristics to Scale Responses and Classifications of Homes. During the three years of study, 239 elderly patients entered the study and completed assessments after being in the homes for one month. Most (85%) had come directly from hospitals and had never been institutionalized before. Average age of the patients was 77 years with a standard deviation of 10 years. Fifty-one percent were male and 18 percent were married currently. Almost all (94%) were white. Last grade completed in school averaged 10 years with a standard deviation of four years. Weekly income averaged about $139 from all sources, and about half had been living alone before placement. None of the patient characteristics were associated significantly with their responses to the scales at one month. Only one characteristic differed across the four classifications of quality. Patients in homes judged as poor were significantly of lower social class than those in excellent homes. However, social class itself was not correlated significantly with scale responses. Because characteristics of the patients were not related to their responses, the analyses comparing responses among the four groups of homes were performed without covariance.

Comparison of Quality of Home Groups by Patient Responses Concerning Activities of Nursing Staff. Table 1 shows mean responses of the patients in the homes grouped by their quality ratings. The overall multivariate difference among the four quality nursing home groups was statistically significant ($p < .05$), with five of the six items showing statistically significant differences at univariate levels. The direction of the

TABLE 1

PATIENTS' RATINGS OF NURSING STAFF BY QUALITY OF HOMES

ITEMS[+]	HOMES				F RATIOS
	Excellent	Good	Fair	Poor	
Treated with Respect by Nursing Staff	2.0	2.2	3.2	3.7	4.9**
Nursing Staff Like Their Work	2.8	2.8	3.9	4.7	5.0**
Someone from NH Staff Special	2.6	3.2	3.8	4.9	4.0**
How Soon Someone Comes When Called	3.1	3.2	4.0	4.3	3.2*
Nursing Home Staff Like You	2.2	1.9	2.9	3.7	3.4*
Someone from Nursing Staff to Talk to	3.4	3.6	3.9	4.8	1.0
Multivariate F					2.5*

*p · .05; **p · .01

[+]Items scored from 1 to 5, with higher score the less favorable response.

mean responses were in the expected directions with less favorable patient responses found in the poor quality homes and the most favorable responses in the homes judged to give excellent quality of care. Three items discriminated at the .01 level among the groups: feeling that nursing staff treated you with respect, liked their work, and having at least one staff member who was special to you. Two items discriminated at the .05 level of significance: how soon calls were answered and feeling liked by the nurses. One item did not discriminate significantly between groups and was relatively high in regard to being unfavorable in all groups: having someone to talk with from the staff. In fact, having some special and someone to talk with was rated a mean of 4.9 (the most unfavorable possible response was 5) by patients in homes judged to be poor. Likewise, poor quality homes were often judged by patients to have nursing staff that did not like their work (rating of 4.7 out of possible 5). Therefore, patients were able to discriminate significantly between homes judged to be of different quality in regard to their perceptions of nursing staff.

Comparison of Quality of Home Groups by Patient Responses About Beliefs of How Nurses Would Behave in Their Nursing Homes in Specific Situations. Table 2 shows the percent of patients choosing the "best" answer to the three situations in each of the four quality of care groups. The multivariate difference was significant at $p < .001$. The greatest difference was found to be related to what the nurses would do if the patient wanted to know more about his physical condition. In the homes judged to provide excellent care, 68% of the patients said the nurse would approach the patient and find out how ill he was feeling compared with only 16% who chose that answer in the homes assessed as giving poor care ($p < .001$). Patient responses in the four groups of homes different at the .01 level in regard to what

TABLE 2

PATIENTS' RATINGS OF BELIEFS ABOUT HOW NURSES BEHAVE

IN THEIR NURSING HOME BY QUALITY OF HOMES

ITEMS[+]	HOMES				F RATIOS
	Excellent	Good	Fair	Poor	
If Patient is Angry:					
Mention the anger and ask if can help	.55	.42	.25	.16	5.2**
Sometimes People Feel Punished by God:					
Encourage patient to talk about feelings	.36	.22	.11	.15	3.2*
Patient Wants to Know More about Physical Condition:					
Approach the patient and find out how ill he is feeling	.68	.44	.34	.16	7.5***
Multivariate F					3.8***

*p < .05; **p < .01; ***p < .001

[+]Items scored No = 0, Yes = 1 (can be read as % by disregarding decimals) the nurse would do if a patient was angry, with 55% in the excellent homes and again only 16% in the poor quality homes saying that the nurse would mention the anger and ask if there was any way the nurse could help. In response to what nurses would do if the patient felt punished for the illness, the differences between patients in the four groups were significant at $p < .05$, with only about a third in the excellent rated group saying patients would be encouraged to talk about their feelings to a low of only 11% in the homes considered as fair quality. Therefore, the majority in all groups indicated the nurse would block further communication about the patient's feelings. In fact, in all of the groups, a large proportion of responses from patients showed that nurses would not encourage communications about anger or feelings about being responsible for one's illness.

DISCUSSION

The major finding in this study was that patients were able to discriminate significantly between nursing homes judged to provide different levels of quality of care within one month after placement into the homes. Those patients in homes judged to provide the highest levels of care reported more favorable perceptions of nursing staff members and their responses to behavioral situations, and those in nursing homes judged to provide lower quality of care reported less favorable perceptions of nursing staff. It would seem, therefore, that the subjective assessments made by professionals familiar with the homes agreed with the experiences of new residents of the home, even though the residents were only asked to evaluate the nursing staff. It is likely that patients formed an overall impression of their environment soon after admission, and the global nature of this impression was reflected in high correlations between their responses to questions dealing with their evaluation of the nursing staff, and it is likely that their responses about the staff would also correlate with other aspects of care. Nursing staff members provide the most frequent source of encounters for patients in nursing homes, and much of their satisfaction with care is probably associated with the outcome of these encounters. The fact that the two subjective sources of evaluation agreed tends to confirm the findings regarding quality of the homes and suggests that residents' reactions to staff members need to be included in assessing quality of care in nursing homes. It also supports the wisdom of encouraging patient participation in activities such as residents' councils in nursing homes as a means of improving quality of care.

Specific responses to the questions suggest that the greatest problems in the poorer homes were associated with suppression of the patients' feelings and open communication. Patients in the homes assessed as poor quality ones believed that the nursing staff would not encourage patients to express angry feelings and would not want them to ask about their illness. In addition, those in the poorest quality homes perceived the nursing staff to be less satisfied with their work than patients in nursing homes judged to provide higher quality of care. Lack of meaningful relationships, staff impersonalization, and lack of encouragement of expression of feelings can produce alienating effects. Other studies[26] have found that staff members sometimes patronize patients by talking down to them and treating them as children, or that complaints about staff members are not taken seriously. Such a climate can alter a patient's self-worth, and ultimately the patients accept the values of the system and in time also perceive themselves as worthless and dependent.

Often satisfaction with care scales elicit answers that are mostly favorable, therefore such scales have not been very useful in discriminating between levels of care in hospital studies. In this study, the questions were related to specific behaviors to staff and were ones that patients could not easily distinguish the most favorable responses. This may have accounted for the rather unfavorable level of responses that were obtained. Even in the good and excellent homes, such items as having someone on the staff with whom they could talk and coming quickly in response to calls had mean scores that were in the unfavorable range of the scale. Certainly, the daily pressures on nursing home staff members, especially aides, to complete routine but necessary tasks in an efficient manner does not leave much time for intimacy and closeness. However, the needs of the patients must be considered. Patients in nursing homes may be very willing and able to provide information to evaluating teams about deficiencies in provision of care. Kane and associates,[27] concerned with assessing outcomes of nursing home patients, emphasized the importance of gathering evaluation data from the nursing home residents themselves. They concluded that it was possible to obtain valid data from nursing home residents. Experiences and results from the present study support the value of soliciting feedback from patients in long-term care facilities.

The only item that did not differentiate between homes was having someone from staff to talk with. Meaningful relationships were notably absent for patients in the 10 facilities. Even those nurses who were perceived by staff to like their work and to come quickly when called to a patient's room will still not have much time to talk if the necessary work gets done.

Although implicit ratings were used in this study, the field of quality assessment has grown so that it is now necessary to examine many areas of care in detail in order to know where specific deficiencies exist. Evaluating care in nursing homes requires consideration of some areas that are not necessarily needed when acute or outpatient care is being assessed. In nursing homes, quality of life issues are extremely important because the nursing home will probably be the person's home for a long period of time. People enter nursing homes for a variety of reasons, such as illness, confusion, disability, social isolation, inability to care for oneself, or a combination of factors. Although the nursing home residents' needs also vary depending upon whether goals of treatment are rehabilitation, management of physical or mental illness, terminal care, or other treatment goals, most residents have a common core of needs. Their needs are for medical services, nursing care, emotional support, personal care, social interaction, a comfortable environment, nutritious and tasty food, cleanliness and safety, information about their health status, contact with the community, and opportunities for privacy, personal choices, and personal growth. Nursing staff members will be the primary providers who can insure that these needs are met.

Helping staff in nursing homes become more aware of the needs of their residents and the fact that answering these needs goes beyond their duties of keeping patients clean and tending only to their body needs appears to be warranted.

In-service training programs or seminars designed to emphasize needs of patients could be helpful. Unlike acute hospitals
with academic affiliation, most nursing homes lack an atmosphere of professional stimulation which arises from contact
with other professional disciplines and students. There is,
however, a growing body of evidence which suggests that
workshops, which are designed to draw on past experiences of
participants, can be potent motivators for change in patient
care practices. Since the bulk of patient care is provided by
nursing staff, greater emphasis must also be placed on recruit-
ment and retention, staffing patterns, job performance, learning needs, and effects of training, especially for nurses aides.

Today there is greater emphasis than ever before on developing a motivating environment[28] for nursing home personnel
and of finding ways to evaluate nursing services.[29] No sector
of health care has been as isolated from the usual rewards,
supports, and sanctions as the nursing home.[30] Nursing home
employees are said to need a lot of recognition since the
services they provide often yield no tangible product that
others can examine and evaluate. Good supervision, involvement in decision-making, and instituting the potential for
change to avoid a deadly routine all can contribute to enrich-
ing the milieu for staff and patients.[28]

There are those[31,32] who strongly urge that nursing homes
become teaching nursing homes through affiliations with academic institutions and hospitals. As places for initial clinical
experience, nursing homes have been said[33] to offer the advantages of having stability of client population, availability of
clients at different points on the health-illness continuum, and
a relatively slower pace. Some factors which have mitigated
against developing long-term care facilities as teaching centers
have been pointed out by Steel and Williams[34] and include
prejudice against the elderly, the acute-oriented medical cur-
riculum, the political system of medical institutions, and the
complexities of caring for the elderly with multiple problems
for which there are no easy solutions. One of the most cogent
arguments in favor of geriatric medicine, along with a brief
history of its development, was provided by Libow[32] who
stated, "So, too, the nursing home will move away from its
major image as a place to die and to die poorly. It has already
become a focus of society's ethical issues and economic dis-

tress. It will evolve as a place respected for treating people, not parts."

Emphasis on training to help members of the nursing staff become sensitive to their patients' feelings and psychological needs and to develop appropriate interpersonal interventions could improve patient satisfaction and raise the quality of care provided. Maintenance of the patients' worth, dignity, and individuality are primary goals. Recognizing a resident's worth and dignity places responsibility on care givers and evaluators to include the residents in the treatment planning and evaluation process. Many nursing home patients can and will give appropriate feedback if given the opportunity.

REFERENCES

1. Kahn KA, Hines W, Woodson AS, et al.: A multidisciplinary approach to assessing the quality of care in long-term care facilities. *Gerontologist* 17:61–65, 1977.

2. Lawton MP: Assessment, integration, and environments for older people. *Gerontologist* 10:38–46, 1970.

3. Linn MW, Gurel L, Linn BS: Patient outcome as a measure of quality of nursing home care. *Am J Public Health* 67:337–344, 1977.

4. Beck P: Two successful interventions in nursing homes: the therapeutic effects of cognitive activity. *Gerontologist* 22:378–383, 1982.

5. Liu K, Manton KG: The characteristics and utilization pattern of an admission cohort of nursing home patients. *Gerontologist* 24:70–76, 1984.

6. Manton KG, Woodbury MS, Liu K: Life tables methods for assessing the dynamics of US nursing home utilization: 1976–1977. *J Gerontol* 39:79–87, 1984.

7. Kane R, Solomon D, Beck J, et al.: The future need for geriatric manpower in the United States. *N Engl J Med* 302:1327–1332, 1980

8. Banziger G, Roush S: Nursing homes for the birds: a control-relevant intervention with bird feeders. *Gerontologist* 23:527–531, 1983.

9. Montgomery RSV: Impact of institutional care policies on family integration. *Gerontologist* 22:54–58, 1982.

10. Shuttlesworth GE, Rubin S, Duffy M: Family versus institutions: incongruent role expectations in the nursing home. *Gerontologist* 22:200–208, 1982.

11. Kane RL, Bell R, Riegler S, et al.: Predicting the outcomes of nursing home patients. *Gerontologist* 23:200–206, 1983.

12. Lieberman MA, Tobin SS: *The Experience of Old Age—Stress, Coping, Survival.* New York, Basic Books, Inc., 1983.

13. Simms LM, Jones SJ, Yoder KK: Adjustment of older persons in nursing homes. *J Gerontological Nurs* 8:383–386, 1982.

14. Townsend P: *The Last Refuge.* London, Routledge & Kegan Paul, 1962.

15. Beattie WM, Bullock J: Evaluating services and personnel in facilities for the aged. In: Leeds M, Shore H (eds), *Geriatric Institutional Management.* New York, Putnam, 1964.

16. Anderson NN, Holmberg RH, Schneider RE, et al.: Policy issues regarding nursing homes: findings from a Minnesota survey. Minneapolis, Institute for Interdisciplinary Studies, American Rehabilitation Foundation, 1969.

17. Levey S, Ruchlin HS, Stotsky BA: An appraisal of nursing home care. *J Gerontol* 28:222–228, 1973.

18. Gottesman LE: Nursing home performance as related to resident traits, ownership, size and source of payment. *Am J Public Health* 64:269–276, 1974.

19. Kosberg JI: Making institutions accountable: research and policy issues. *Gerontologist* 14:510–516, 1974.

20. Linn MW, Gurel L, Linn BS: Patient outcome as a measure of quality of nursing home care. *Am J Public Health* 87:337–344, 1977.

21. Linn MW, Gurel L, Williford WO, et al.: Nursing home care as an alternative to psychiatric hospitalization. *Arch Gen Psychiatry* 42:544–551, 1985.

22. White KL: Evaluation of medical education and health care. In: Lathem, Willoughby, Newberry A (eds), *Community Medicine: Teaching, Research and Health Care.* New York, Appleton-Century-Crofts, 1970.

23. Linn MW: Predicting quality of care in nursing homes. *Gerontologist* 14:225–227, 1974.

24. Linn MW: A nursing home rating scale. *Geriatrics* 21:188–192, 1966.

25. Bancroft TA: Topics in intermediate statistical methods. Ames, IA, Iowa State University Press, 1968.

26. Mercer S, Kane RA: Helplessness and hopelessness among the institutionalized aged: an experiment. *Health Soc Work* 4:90–115, 1979.

27. Kane RL, Bell R, Riegler S, et al.: Assessing the outcomes of nursing home patients. *J Gerontol* 38:385–393, 1983.

28. Gordon GK: Developing a motivating environment. *J Nurs Adm* 12:11–16, 1982.

29. Bloch D: Evaluation of nursing care in terms of process and outcome: issues in research and quality assurance. *Nurs Res* 24:256–263, 1975.

30. Mezey M: Implications for the health professions. *Geriatr Nurs* 4:241–244, 1983.

31. Mezey MD, Lynaugh JE, Cherry JE: The teaching nursing home program. *Nurs Outlook* 32:146–150, 1984.

32. Libow LS: Geriatric medicine and the nursing home: a mechanism for mutual excellence. *Gerontologist* 22:134–141, 1982.

33. Neil R, Casey T, Kennedy MA: Nursing homes for initial clinical experience: some specific advantages. *Nurs Health Care* 3:319–323, 1982.

34. Steel K, Williams TF: Geriatrics. "Fruition of the clinician." *Arch Intern Med* 134:1125–1126, 1974.

Is Laughter the Best Medicine?
A Study of the Effects
of Humor on Perceived
Pain and Affect

Elizabeth R. Adams
Francis A. McGuire

ABSTRACT. This paper presents a study of the effects of humor on affect and perceived pain in elderly residents of a long-term care facility. Movies were viewed by two groups (humor and non-humor) and differences between groups were noted on measures of perceived pain and affect. Humor is shown to provide significant benefits to aged clients. Qualitative information on program implementation is included.

In keeping with modern concepts of holistic medicine and body awareness, it is assumed that there is a complex system of exchanges between psychological and physiological processes. Laughter is an observable reaction to a humorous situation in which physiologically, "muscles are activated; heart rate is increased; respiration is amplified, with increase in oxygen exchange . . ." (Fry, 1971). Psychologically, laughter is inconsistent with anger which can precipitate heart attacks. It is also inconsistent with depression, which has been suggested as a factor in the onset of cancer.

The fact that laughter makes people feel better can be verified by many nurses at long-term care facilities, and humor as therapy is enjoying a surge of interest as evidenced by the recent formation of the organization Nurses for Laughter (whose leader is known as the Master Giggler). These nurses

---

The authors are affiliated with the Department of Parks, Recreation and Tourism Management, Clemson University, Clemson, SC.

are "committed to promoting the use of humor in nursing homes and health care. . . ."

There has been an increase in the number of studies using humor as an experimental variable, primarily in the field of psychoanalysis (Goldstein and McGhee, 1972). Historically, humor has played a major role in the mental health field (Chapman and Foot, 1977). Freud's extensive analysis of the joke and the human psyche contributes to the perception of humor as a very important aspect of human nature. [This, coupled with the new awareness of mind and body correspondence, leads us to anticipate benefits of laughter in patients who experience pain as a symptom of disease or disorders as well as those who suffer from emotional difficulties.]

An article by L. Rhodes (1983) entitled "Laughter and Suffering: Sinhalese Interpretations of the Use of Ritual Humor" describes the use of humor in exorcising psychological factors thought to cause pain. In Sri Lanka, it is believed that laughter purifies the blood and the body and relieves the sufferer of demon-induced discomfort. It is a mystical interpretation of pain and is aligned with the concept of pain as a stress-related phenomenon.

It terms of the aged population, pain perception is aggravated by long spans of idleness. According to Miller and Le-Lieuvre (1982) " . . . older people have more time to think of their physical condition and to become preoccupied with pain. They also may receive attention and other reinforcers from sympathetic persons for complaining of the pain." Therefore, the reduction of unoccupied time may result in decreased perceptions of pain by the elderly. The physical benefits of laughter combine with the psychological effects of alleviation of boredom.

One of the most frequently reported health symptoms of the elderly is pain. Many illnesses associated with aging, such as arthritis, are accompanied by frequent and persistent pain. Older people have time to think about their physical condition and to become preoccupied with pain (Miller and Le-Lieuvre, 1982). This manifests itself in problems of discomfort, but furthermore, activity is sharply decreased when pain is present. It is the primary reason for decline in activity among the elderly (Brody and Kleban, 1983). There is a need for examining ways of reducing pain and its debilitating effects for the aged population.

Medication is the treatment most commonly used in reducing pain. Changing and often unidentified reactions to medication are especially problematical in the elderly where multiple drugs are often being used. It is probable that older individuals are at a greater risk when medication is the sole intervention for controlling pain (Miller and LeLieuvre, 1982). Other possible treatments for pain reduction that do not carry the risks of chemical analgesics must be identified.

A largely unexplored area is the use of the body's own healing powers. Norman Cousins, in his book *The Anatomy of an Illness as Perceived by the Patient* (1979), reports his success in using humor and laughter in reducing pain. Cousins based his work on the belief that there is a close link between the mind and body and that this interaction could be either positive or negative. His findings indicate that positive emotions may produce positive chemical changes effective in combatting pain. A possible explanation for this finding is provided by Dubos (1979). There exist in the body a group of hormones known as endorphins. The physiological actions of endorphins are similar to those of morphine and other opiate substances which relieve pain. According to Henry (1982) endorphins evoke a feeling of well-being and serve as an analgesia. An alternative explanation is that laughter serves in reducing stress, and thereby stress-related diseases and associated pain.

The therapeutic effects of humor have long been recognized, and laughter is generally accepted as the best medicine. However, what is generally accepted is not always the basis for planning therapeutic recreation activities. In order to foster a more receptive climate for laughter in long-term care facilities, this paper reports the findings of an empirical study which concerns the relationships among humor, affect, and perceived pain. Specifically, the following hypotheses were tested in this study:

1. Individuals viewing humorous movies will experience more reduction in perceived pain than individuals viewing non-humorous movies;

2. Individuals viewing humorous movies will experience more improvement in affect than individuals viewing non-humorous movies.

Due to the exploratory nature of this study, and a resulting hesitancy to risk a Type II error and conclude there is no effect of humor when in fact there is one, the .10 level of significance was used to test hypotheses rather than a more conservative .05.

METHODOLOGY

The subjects chosen for this study were residents of a long term care facility in South Carolina. Individuals were selected on the basis of the following criteria: (a) chronic pain and requests for pain medication; (b) no scheduled medical or surgical procedure; (c) interest in participating in the study and completing all required human subject procedures. The proposed design provided for three groups of ten subjects each. One group was to view humorous movies, one group to view non-humorous movies, and one group to act as a control group. Although use of a control group acts as a strengthening feature in experimental design, ethical considerations precluded withholding treatment from persons wishing to participate. Therefore, the final design consisted of two groups: one group with humorous treatment; and one group with non-humorous treatment.

The participants were invited to view movies on videotape, a medium selected for economic and practical reasons. The use of video facilitated dividing the films into three segments of approximately thirty minutes each, a time span well within the range of attention of the participants. The segments were shown on three subsequent days of each week, and the program lasted for six weeks. The treatment was scheduled for subsequent days in order to eliminate unnecessary time intervals that may have allowed the participants to forget the story line of the movies. Two locations were provided by the long term care facility, and as these locations differed in spatial and lighting considerations, the groups alternated weeks in each location. This eliminated the effects of the specific location, and the effects of mobility to and from the location. The facility is situated on two floors necessitating elevator trips for some of the participants. Two researchers also alternated groups, thus eliminating the effects of a particular personality on the results.

Movies were selected by the researchers. However, after the first film, the tastes of the residents became apparent and were subsequently taken into consideration. Older movies were preferred, and care was taken that the humorous and the non-humorous films shown in the same week were either both in color or both in black and white. A short warm-up discussion consisted of jokes for the humor group, and informal talk of a general nature for the non-humor group.

The groups grew and shrank during the program as some participants' enthusiasm for the movies spread to their neighbors and as others dropped out. However, enough of the original groups remained at the end for statistical measures to be seriously considered (humor group, n = 7; non-humor group, n = 6).

RESULTS

The instruments chosen to measure perceived pain was the McGill Pain Assessment Questionnaire. This self-reporting device relies upon a comprehensive list of descriptive words divided into categories of pain experiences. In that it is comprehensive, it is also lengthy. To properly administer the instrument, the entire list must be read and evaluated by the participants. Difficulty in accomplishing this lead to a decision to evaluate the pain perceptions of the patients subjectively, and therefore, the hypothesis related to humor and pain was not statistically tested. The resulting comments made by the patients must therefore be viewed in the light of their subjective nature and the desire of the patients to please the researchers, which after six weeks of contact was a delightful and unanticipated outcome of the research. The fact that most participants claimed to feel less pain at the end of the program must be left to the realm of judgment and belief on the part of the reader.

A second measure of pain was obtained through the examination of the medical charts of participants. At the conclusion of the study, the charts of each subject were examined, and the amount of medication taken every day of the study was calculated. The accompanying figures may be taken as an indication of the effectiveness of the program. The observations represent the total number of PRN medications taken by an individual during each of two baseline weeks prior to the beginning of the study and during the six weeks of the study. A visual scan of the figures will reveal a decrease in PRN medications for every member of the humor group taking medication (see Figures 1a-e). Not so decisive are the figures of subjects in the non-humor group (see Figures 2a-e). While some members of this group did experience a decrease in medication, others did not. This implies that treatment of a non-humorous nature may or may not be an effective means of decreasing perceived pain, while treatment of a humorous type more definitively does decrease perceived pain.

Affect was measured using the Affect Balance Scale (ABS) which was developed by Bradburn (1969). Affect is defined as a global feeling toward life in the present, and the ABS asks individuals to indicate whether they have experienced specific feelings, both positive and negative, in the past few weeks. The ABS is the best available measure of affect (George and Bearon, 1980). The ABS was administered to study participants one week before the initiation of the program of movies and one week after its conclusion. Data from the ABS were used to test the hypothesis related to humor and affect.

Data analysis indicated the subjects viewing humorous movies did not differ from those viewing non-humorous movies on pre-test ABS scores (Mann-Whitney U = 20.5, p = .9413). Comparisons of the pre-test and post-test scores, based on the Wilcoxon Matched Pairs Signed Ranks Test, of the humor group and non-humor group indicated that both experienced significant improvements in affect over the course of the study (p = .04 for both groups). Comparison of the post-test scores of the two groups indicated that the individuals viewing humorous movies had significantly higher affect scores than individuals viewing non-humorous movies (U = 14.0, 1-tailed p = .08). Therefore, hypothesis 2 was accepted.

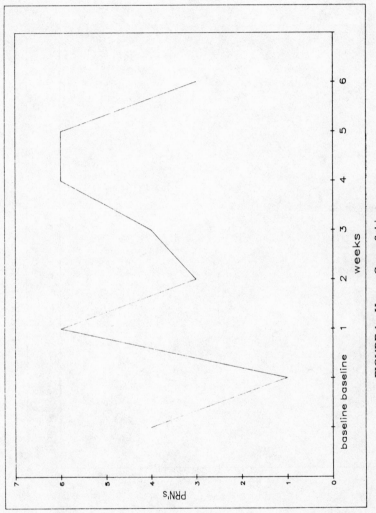

FIGURE 1a: Humor Group Subject

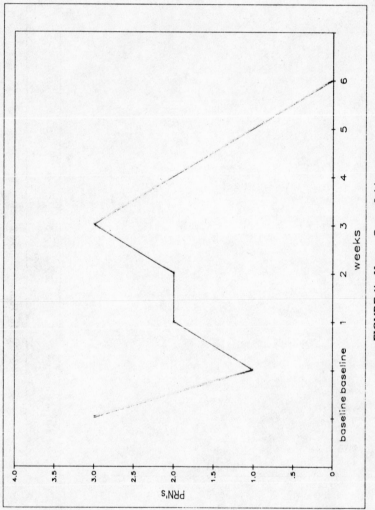

FIGURE 1b: Humor Group Subject

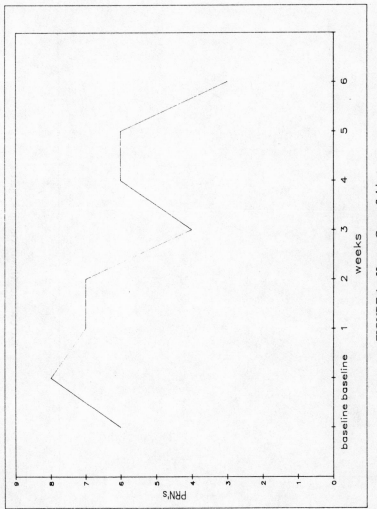

FIGURE 1c: Humor Group Subject

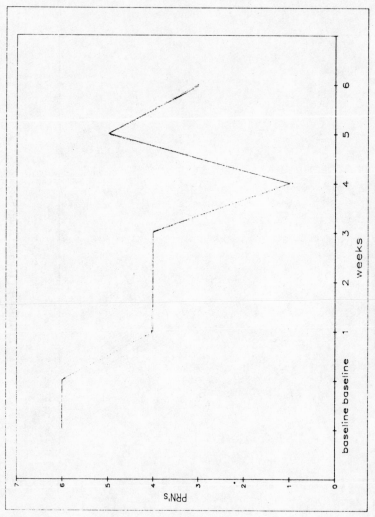

FIGURE 1d: Humor Group Subject

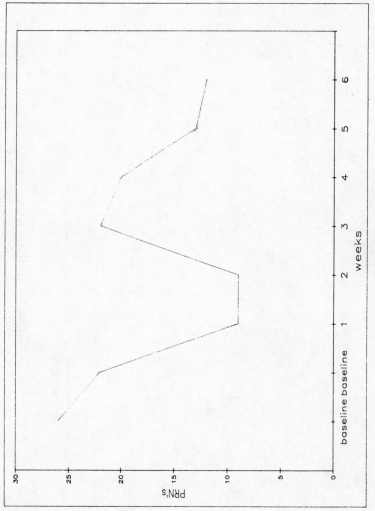

FIGURE 1e: Humor Group Subject

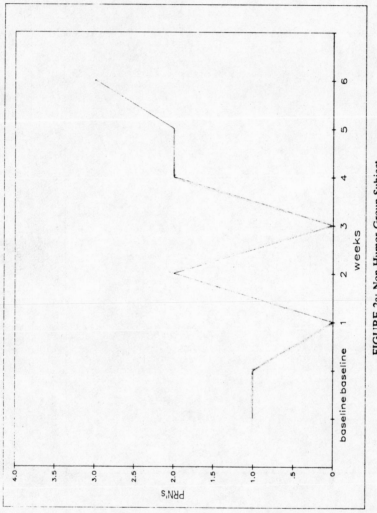

FIGURE 2a: Non-Humor Group Subject

168

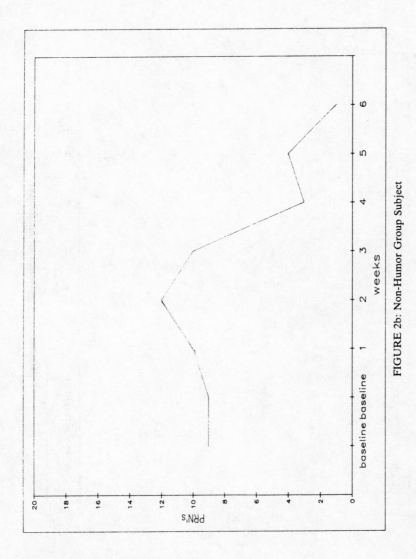

FIGURE 2b: Non-Humor Group Subject

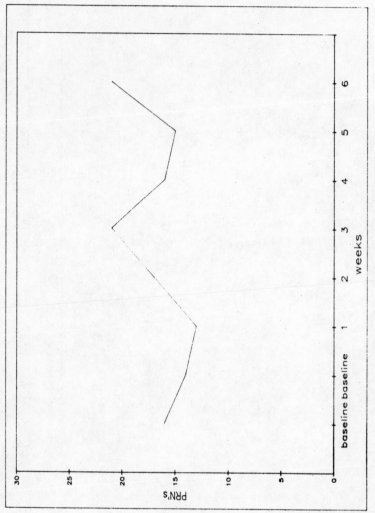

FIGURE 2c: Non-Humor Group Subject

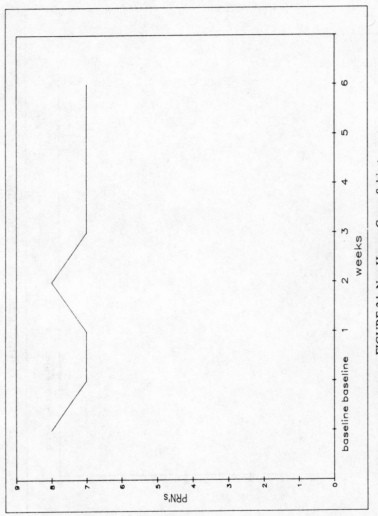

FIGURE 2d: Non-Humor Group Subject

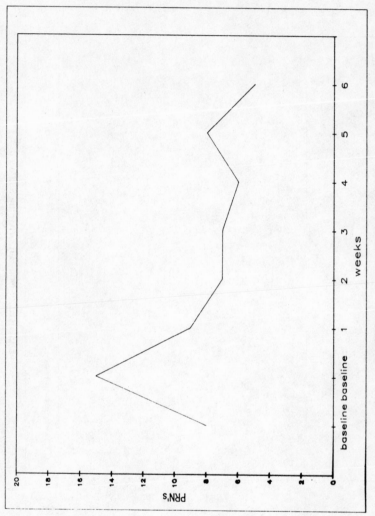

FIGURE 2e: Non-Humor Group Subject

DISCUSSION

In the interest of broadening research perspectives in the social sciences, certain qualitative observations follow which were made during the study. These may be useful to researchers who wish to expand upon the use of humor as therapy, as well as to practitioners anxious to impart the benefits of humor to their clients.

When showing films to older individuals, some modifications may be in order. The use of a large viewing screen will be helpful for those with visual limitations. When television screens and VCRs are mandated by financial considerations, small groups will ensure that everyone has a good view. This is especially the case when many participants are confined to wheelchairs which take up more room than ordinary chairs.

Our viewers responded most favorably to visual, slapstick humor. Many were suffering from impairments which affected their attention spans and their ability to react to complicated story lines and verbal jokes. Abbott and Costello got the best reviews, in general. However, the most prolonged and hearty laughter was in response to Marilyn Monroe's performance in "How to Marry a Millionaire." Blind as a bat, she walked into walls with her glasses.

The participants responded as much to the researchers as to the movies themselves. It is recommended that warm-up jokes be told prior to the movies. Also, staff members known to possess infectuous laughs themselves should be invited to come and trigger laughter in the clients.

Movies should be previewed. Especially in older populations, anything likely to be seen as offensive may negate the benefits of the treatment. One of our participants quit the study because of Henry Fonda's mild profanity in "On Golden Pond." Older movies are more meaningful to most older people, and are usually morally stringent. For these reasons, when available, older movies should be shown to older people.

With respect to attention span, our dividing each movie and showing the segments on subsequent days had no adverse effects. Many people in our sample could not attend or sit comfortably for longer periods. Continuity across days was not an important factor in that laughter was invoked by gags that would be funny even taken completely out of context. Some patients expressed disappointment when shorter films were stopped after twenty minutes (in contrast to the usual thirty).

Occasionally, a patient would talk or mumble during the movie, distracting others in the group. This caused problems at times, as we let anyone stay who wished to do so. Perhaps, as a practical consideration, such people could be treated separately.

The staff of the facility was instrumental in transporting patients, particularly those in wheelchairs, to and from their appropriate locations, thus simplifying what was not foreseen as a complication. Their encouragement to the participants was also invaluable, as many residents were loathe to leave their rooms for any reason.

A full program of humor has been instituted by the Ethel Percy Andrus Gerontology Center with great success. Their handbook on program development using humor contains a wealth of information that will interest caregivers in long-term care facilities (Ewers, Jacobson, Powers, and McConney, 1983).

The improvement in the quality of life for the participants as indicated by these results points to the need for more and better programming for residents of long term care facilities. Recreational programs are beneficial; this is evident. However, programs promoting humor and laughter are even more so.

REFERENCES

Bradburn, N.M. *The structure of psychological well-being.* Chicago: Aldine, 1969.

Brody, E.M. & Kleban, M.H. Day-to-day mental and physical health symptoms of older people: A report on health logs. *The Gerontologist,* 1983, *23,* 75–85.

Chapman, A.J. & Foot, H.C. *It's a funny thing, humour.* Oxford: Pergamon Press, 1977.

Cousins, N. *Anatomy of an illness as perceived by the patient.* Toronto: Bantam Books, 1979.

Dubos, R. In introduction to Cousins, N. *Anatomy of an illness as perceived by the patient.* Toronto: Bantam Books, 1979.

Ewers, M., Jacobson, S., Powers, V., McConney, P. & Krauss, I. *Humor: The tonic you can afford.* Los Angeles: University of Southern California, 1983.

Freud, S. *Jokes and their relation to the unconscious.* New York: W. W. Norton & Co., 1960.

Fry, W. F. Laughter: Is it the best medicine? *Stanford M.D.*, Winter 1971, *10*, 16–20.

George, L.K. & Bearon, L.B. *Quality of life in older persons: Meanings and measurement.* New York: Human Sciences Press, 1980.

Goldstein, J.H. & McGhee, P.E. *The psychology of humor.* New York: Academic Press, 1972.

Henry, J.L. Circulating opiods: Possible physiological roles in central nervous system function. *Neuroscience and Biobehavioral Review*, 1982, *6*, 229–245

Melzack, R. The McGill pain questionnaire: Major properties and scoring methods. *Pain.* Amsterdam: Elsevier/North-Holland, 1975.

Miller, C. & LeLieuvre, R.B. A method to reduce chronic pain in elderly nursing home residents. *The Gerontologist*, 1982, *22*, 314–317.

Rhodes, Lorna A. Laughter and suffering: Sinhalese interpretations of the use of ritual humor. *Social Science & Medicine*, 1983, 17, 979–984.

The Interface of Activity and Psychopharmacological Agents

Leon Hyer
Richard Bagge

ABSTRACT. Older age psychiatric patients are not often viewed as part of the life span developmental process. They are treated conservatively and "educated" to reduce active life styles. A social breakdown syndrome often results. This article argues that better care among the elderly psychiatric patients often involves both psychopharmacological and psychosocial interventions. Commonly, the latter suffers at the hands of the former. This is due largely to myths, staff bias or prepotent staff management needs, as well as poor care in general. The goal of older age psychiatric care could be autonomy and independence even among frail psychiatric elders. On this behalf, a simple schema of psychopharmacologic agents and side effects, five psychopharmacologic and psychosocial principles, and a "Treatment Autonomy Schema," are offered.

Psychiatric treatment of later life problems is a new and challenging area. While there is still debate about this topic, treatment generally involves methods and techniques distinct from those applied at younger ages (Birren & Sloan, 1980; Brink, 1977). Therapists who treat older people are often required to be more active, to manage, and even to be an advocate for patients. Traditional therapy is often less appropriate.

One reason for this alteration in treatment style involves the therapeutic necessity for intervention in many areas of a patient's life. This often involves an admixture of psychopharmacologic agents and psychosocial interventions. The interaction of these two treatment types with older people is little

---

Leon Hyer, EdD, is with the VA Medical Center, Augusta, GA, and the Medical College of Georgia. Richard Bagge, MD is also with the Medical College of Georgia. Please address inquiries to: Leon Hyer, Psychology Service (116BU), 2460 Wrightsboro Rd. (10), Augusta, GA 30910.

understood and often a problem for both therapist and patient. From the research literature, there are few solid outcome studies comparing types of treatment with older people (Levy et al., 1980). There is, however, every indication that older people do respond well to selected types of psychosocial interventions (Gottesman, 1980; Sparacino, 1981; Wellerman & McCormick, 1984; Willner, 1978) *and* to psychopharmacologic agents (Blazer, 1982; Hicks et al., 1980; Whanger, 1980). This interface is often confusing, often little understood, and often a problem.

The purpose of this article is to provide a better understanding for the dynamic relationship between psychopharmacologic *and* psychosocial treatment with older people. This is not a how-to manual. Rather, this paper is intended to isolate important principles of both treatment types. First, an overview of activity as an index of treatment in later life is presented. Second, a drug classification scheme is provided with a focus on the potential side effects. Finally, treatment rules are given for the care of older patients who are required to take medications. An intervention/activity schema is also added. At a higher level, this article attempts to undermine the "social breakdown syndrome" (Bengsten, 1973), and to provide an optimistic (but realistic) appraisal of later life pathology. This article then, argues for growth and independent functioning as the key or guide in therapy, even among the frail elderly. This concept is regarded as *the* central principle of later life treatment.

OVERVIEW OF ACTIVITY

During the past decade there has been an explosion in the research literature noting the change in older age functioning. There has evolved a conceptual shift in later life problems; a "regression hypothesis" has yielded to a "growth hypothesis" (Hyer, Tamkin, Barry & McConatha, 1984). Except when the focus is on the frail elderly, normal older people cope (Lazarus & Delongis, 1983), enjoy (Flannigan, 1978), and behave (Birren, 1983), as well or better than at other ages. The more popular models of human development (e.g., the life span developmental model) have advocated continuous growth and change. Crises are no longer considered pathological or even problematic. Problems are as likely to result in positive outcomes, as otherwise. Given this view, the goal behind treatment interventions is not only to prevent crises, but to enhance or enrich abilities to deal constructively with these so as to cause growth in other life areas (Danish & D'Augelli, 1980).

This creative and "fanning out" process (Neugarten, 1979), however, becomes truncated when frail or problem laden elders are considered. This occurs for a variety of reasons, both intrinsic to the illness and secondary to it. Physical illness is a fact of life at later ages, with greater than 70% above the age of 65 being afflicted with at least one major medical problem (Storandt, 1983). When this occurs, the possibility of mental problems is increased, usually reactively based and transient, but painful none-the-less.

A natural concomitant of these disorders is a retrenchment of activities. In fact, this appears to be an essential element of mental pathology, as activity is a key factor in life satisfaction (Flannigan, 1978) and a causative element in treatment change (deVries & Adams, 1972; Powell, 1974; Morgan & Pollock, 1976; Wiswell, 1980). While activity in leisure pursuits does decrease with age, it represents a reordering of interests in most cases. Psychiatric patients tend to be less active. Whether due to acute distress or "acute on chronic" distress, these patients often seek the patient role (Maddox, 1973), assume an external locus of control (Wolk & Kurtz, 1975) and a lower sense of well being (Wolk & Telleen, 1976). With the frail elder especially, a reduction in activity seems to represent a final common pathway of illness expression.

A key treatment problem here is that since age and illness are so intertwined, distinctions become blurred and one is excessively influenced by the latter at the expense of the former. Therapeutic caution and defensive treatment often result. This may lead to "custodialism" (Zarit, 1980) or a sort of "new agism" (Kalish, 1982). The health care provider becomes "too impressed" with pathology (Wiswell, 1980) and ignores or defensively treats elders. "Excess disability" results (Brody, 1972). In an institutional setting these iatrogenic problems can become endemic and result in the social breakdown syndrome mentioned earlier.

The judicious use of monitored activity, therefore, is often the best index of change. Behavior modification programs have advocated their position for a long period (Hussain, 1982). Healthy activity, even in the service of a disengagement process, represents adjustment (Anderson, 1967; Neugarten, 1977). Among psychiatric groups, there are two problems, in particular, that benefit from structured activity or exercise: depression (Morgan & Pollock, 1976; Powell, 1974) and dementia (Newsome, 1983; Renner, Eberly & Patterson, 1983). In nursing homes, where upwards of 90% of the residents' time is spent in non-activity (Hussain, 1982), the treatment of choice *becomes* activity; remotivation, recreation and an active reality orientation, as well as activity therapy itself. Bigot (1982) has even employed an activity inventory on 21 activities in nursing homes to isolate and treat types of residents.

It seems clear, then, that activity is an index of pathology, particularly at later life. It is both a final common pathway of pathology and a point of reference for change. The psychological effects of exercise, even minimal exercise on psychiatric problems are well documented (Wiswell, 1980), and for older psychiatric patients, a decline in these areas is most often a function of the pathology and a negative adjustment sign.

PSYCHOPHARMACOLOGICAL PROBLEMS

Psychopharmacological agents are often a major contributant to inactivity among older age people. In recent years, physicians and health care providers in general have become aware of the interactive and dose related effects of psychopharmacologic agents on older people (Poe & Holloway, 1981). It is now common practice for a physician to conduct a drug history and to remove unwarranted medications. It has also become prescription policy to "start low and go slow" with late life problems (Blazer, 1982). In addition, medication education and compliance techniques are increasing among physicians.

One clinically useful taxonomy divides psychopharamcological agents into four types: antidepressants, anxiolytics, antipsychotics, and lithium. Each of these have potential adverse reactions. Most common are: anticholinergic reactions, sedative effects, cardiac reactions, hypotensive reactions (postural), extrapyramidal side effects, impaired motor coordination and tardive dyskinesia. Briefly, these involve:

—*Anticholinergic effects:* blurred vision, dry mouth, constipation, urinary retention, confusion, and possibly psychosis.
—*Sedative effects/impaired motor coordination:* patient sleepiness and decreased attentiveness.
—*Cardiac effects:* arrhythmias and conduction defects, among others; in tricyclic antidepressants, overdosage causes serious problems.
—*Postural hypotension:* dizziness and loss of balance when changing position from a reclining or squatting position to a sitting or standing position.
—*Extrapyramidal side effects:* These include: (1) dystonias, muscle contractions that may occur as facial grimacing, torticollis, occulogyric crisis; (2) akathisias, inner restlessness producing a constant motion; (3) parkinsonism like syndrome: flattening of affect, drooling, tremor, and shuffling gait; and (4) tardive dyskinesia: a late onset movement disorder characterized by stereotyped involuntary movements of the mouth and tongue as well as other muscle groups.

The fact that the elderly are more prone to side effects from medications is well known. It is reported that adverse drug reactions occur seven times more frequently in those over the age of 65 than those among the 20-29 year old group (Crook & Cohen, 1981). This is due to differences in drug response as a result of age. These involve problems due to absorption, distribution, metabolism, excretion, as well as in person-specific responses to the drug. The impact of these side effects on the patient are important in the treatment plans.

Table 1 provides a schema of adverse reactions in older people. Antidepressants are the drugs most frequently used by older people. Elders are most susceptible to side effects of these drugs. As a group, antidepressants influence the norepinephrine and serotonin neurotransmitters. Various subtypes

Table 1

Adverse Reactions By Drug Classification

Drug Class

Side Effects	Antidepressants	Antipsychotics	Axiolytics	Lithium
Anticholinergic	yes	yes	no	no
Sedative	yes	yes	yes	may
Cardiac	yes	yes	no	yes
Postural hypotension	yes	yes	no	no
Extrapyramidal	rare	yes	no	no
Tardive dyskinesia	no	yes	no	no

have differing amounts of anticholinergic side effects. Constipation, in particular, can be quite severe. Drugs high in the anticholinergic effects are often high in sedative actions. If sedation is a short term desirable side effect for the patient, then the patient will be forced to tolerate other adverse reactions. Daytime drowsiness will then be a problem and may be severe enough to warrant discontinuation of the drug. Postural hypotension also is a side effect. This has particular problem potential in the elderly because of increased likelihood of falling and breaking bones. Special precautions are required if this problem develops. Postural blood pressure readings are helpful in spotting potential problems. Finally, cardiac side effects are numerous in the elderly. Arrhythmias and conduction defects, as well as a decreased cardiac output, often result (Bernstein, 1983).

The antipsychotic medications are also used frequently with the elderly. At times these are prescribed simply for patient management and this should only exist for short term use. As a whole, however, older age groups are most sensitive to possible adverse reactions. The low potency drugs, such as chlorpromazine and thioridazine, have more hypotensive effects, sedation, anticholinergic effects and cardiovascular problems. The high potency drugs, such as haloperidol and prolixin, are more likely to cause extrapyramidal side effects; dystonias, akathisias, and a parkinsonian-like syndrome. Both can cause all of these problems, as well as tardive dyskinesia. An added problem of these drugs are medications used to treat the extrapyramidal side effects. Most can cause anticholinergic effects. This adds to the potential for an anticholinergic delirium which may be difficult to differentiate from a psychosis secondary to a dementia.

Anxiolytics are increasingly being used for later life problems. The two most important of these are the benzodiazepines and the antihistamines. The benzodiazepines are sedating drugs and may cause confusion, poor coordination, and on occasion sleeplessness. The major problem with these drugs is the long half-life. This is especially a concern with diazepam (Valium) and chlordiazepoxide (Librium), whose half-life may be double that of an average adult. This can lead to high blood levels in the geriatric patient exacerbating problems, especially organic brain syndrome (e.g., senile dementia). These drugs can also produce paradoxical agitation. With benzodiazepines, it is best to use shorter acting agents, such as lorazepam, oxazepam, or alprazolam. Secondly, it is noted that antihistamines have many of these same effects, especially sedation. A special problem with these drugs is anticholinergic effects.

Lithium is a psychopharmacologic agent that is effective in stabilizing manic problems. It is also helpful in preventing recurrence of depression. Lithium itself is a salt which is eliminated by the kidney. As a person ages, their renal function decreases, resulting in higher levels. A toxic level of lithium can cause severe cardiac problems, coma and even death. Usual side effects include polydipsia and polyuria, nausea, and a fine hand tremor. This last problem may be severe enough to interface with activities of daily living. In general, lower doses of lithium are usually sufficient in the geriatric patient.

TREATMENT RULES

As noted, in recent years health care providers of the elderly with psychiatric problems have been hyper-sensitive to negative effects of psychopharmacologic agents. Polypharmacy (Schmucher, 1984) and tardive dyskenesia (Jenike, 1984), especially, have been recognized as problem areas. In addition, newer psychopharmacological prescription guidelines regarding the elderly have begun to appreciate the value of active life styles (Blazer, 1982; Vieth, 1981). In fact, the concept of titration involves the key requirement of symptom reduction *and* active growth and change. Increasingly, psychopharmacologic regimens of older people prescribe lower dosages, allow for drug holidays, avoid polypharmacy, and advocate an active treatment plan. Both symptom reduction and planned positive behavior change combine for better care.

The authors have isolated five treatment rules that, above all others, apply to the practice of psychopharmacologic and psychosocial treatment of the elderly. These are best viewed as clinical strategies (Goldfried, 1976) that represent good clinical care and treatment goals. They do not preclude many other excellent guidelines for the elderly psychiatric patient. They are:

1. Good psychopharmacological regimes involve a *short term* approach combined with support and counseling. The titration of psychopharmacologic agents and other therapies should not only involve a reduction of negative symptoms of older people (usually anxiety, depression, and paranoid symptoms), but a facilitation of positive signs (behavioral goals and growth oriented objectives where possible). The gradual elimination of medication is a desired goal. Where this cannot be done due to continued symptom presence, lower drug dosages should be attempted.

2. The goal of psychopharmacologic treatment is *autonomy*. Autonomy involves control by the patient, choice by the patient, and involvement by the patient. Staff or family considerations should be secondary to these.

3. Activity among older persons with psychiatric problems can be equated with good mental health. This assumes that activity is a necessary condition for good mental health. It also assumes that healthy activity or active leisure pursuits do not just "happen." These are *learned*. With the elderly especially, activities related to one's lifestyle involve study and opportunity (Meyer, 1983). Health care providers must actively intervene.

4. Although physical health and mental health problems cohabitate, one need not necessarily impede the other. While caution is a consideration, harm is often done in the service of conservative treatment. Harm is a result of treatment programs that foster excessive dependency, inactivity, lack of stimulation, sensory loss and the like. The resources of the older person require assessment. This is a continuous process. Independent functioning is the goal.

5. Whatever the level of dysfunction, task oriented and structural activities are strongly endorsed. This does not have to be a "total push" program. It must, however, reverse the "social breakdown syndrome" and create a psychosocial press for activity and positive change.

No series of principles are ever complete. However, these represent an active, aggressive and positive approach. They also represent an integrative one. The goal is to reduce a dysfunction with the least intrusive intervention and reinforce positive behavior change in the service of autonomy and independence. This is best done in an interactive fashion according to the level of functioning of the patient. A therapeutic armamentarium and active, eclectic approach is best. Basically, this involves a health orientation. More commonly, the alleviation of illness is the focus. This is sickness orientation. Older psychiatric patients require both. Frequently, however, the health side of the equation suffers due to bias, myth, and excessive treatment leading to increased disabilities. Often too, treatments are prescribed for patient control. Manageability can be a problem, especially with highly agitated patients or patients in the later stages of dementia. But, even under these circumstances, treatment related to the facilitation of independence is appropriate. A facilitative environment, titrated medications, and treatment goals related to patient autonomy can be applied.

The rehabilitative step ladder is often a long one for older people. Indeed, it may never end. Often the prevention of further regression or a goal of stabilization is all that can be offered. With the frail elder especially, it is now clear that, even though substantial effort might not result in therapeutic remission, regression almost certainly will result without it (Levy et al., 1980). Erickson (1975) has noted that almost any concerted effort, if judiciously applied and directed to patient autonomy, can result in positive effects. Many efforts may be required with the frail elder.

Figure 1 presents an "Treatment Autonomy schema." This is a heuristic model that specifies treatment efforts—psychopharmacologic agents, psychosocial interventions and environmental input in relation to the patient's level of functioning. When patients are inert or panic laden, higher dosages of medications, a greater, more aggressive "amount" of psychosocial input and more environmental supports are required. As the patient functions better, autonomy increases until little or no medication is required. As this occurs, only educative or growth related therapy is required and little or no environmental assistance is in order. The goal of minimal staff intervention (of all types) and maximal patient self efficacy is achieved. While this schema is most apt for the elder with potential for change, it is applicable to all later life cases, even frail elders.

CONCLUSION

The central thesis of this article is that older age is the culmination of a life span process. This view is not new. When psychiatric problems do occur, the health care provider can be optimistic. As is currently practiced, however, the interface of psychopharmacologic agents and psychosocial treatment is often blurry. Most often, the former is more heavily relied on at the expense of the latter. This occurs because of management needs, family or staff bias, as well as reasons related to poor treatment in general.

It is argued here that the best care is one that fosters independence and autonomy. Psychopharmacologic agents and their side effects were outlined. It is believed that not only can these side effects be reduced but that active growth can occur. Five principles are provided on this behalf. Medication is best used in the service of autonomy. It is argued further that activity and change do not just "happen." These must be learned and opportunities must be provided. Indeed the health care provider of the elder with psychiatric problems is an active agent of change. This requires an armamentarium of many treatment modalities, as well as a good understanding of psychiatric problems and psychopharmacologic agents.

Figure 1

Autonomy Treatment Schema

Psychosocial Interventions

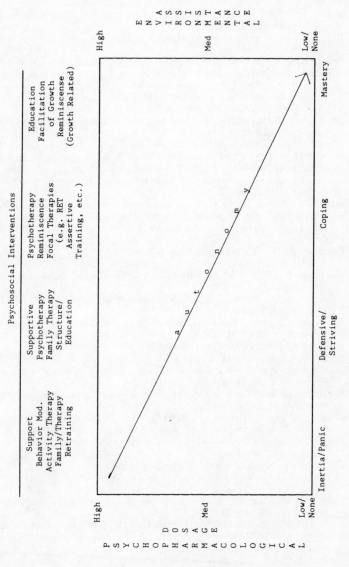

Support	Supportive	Psychotherapy	Education
Behavior Mod.	Psychotherapy	Reminiscence	Facilitation
Activity Therapy	Family Therapy	Focal Therapies	of Growth
Family/Therapy	Structure/	(e.g. RET	Reminiscense
Retraining	Education	Assertive	(Growth Related)
		Training, etc.)	

PSYCHOPATHOLOGY SCALE — High / Med / Low/None

ENVIRONMENTAL STRESS INVOLVEMENT — High / Med / Low/None

autonomy

Inertia/Panic — Defensive/Striving — Coping — Mastery

REFERENCES

Blazer, D. (1982). *Depression in late life.* St. Louis: Mosby.

Birren, Jr. (1983). Aging in America: Roles for psychology, *American Psychologist, 38,* 298–299.

Birren, J. & Sloan, R. (1980). *Handbook of mental health and aging.* Englewood Cliffs, NJ: Prentice Hall.

Bengtson, V. (1973). *The social psychology of aging.* Indianapolis: Bobbs-Merill.

Bernstein, J. (1983). *Handbook of drug therapy in psychiatry.* John Wright PSG.

Bigot, A. (1982). *Research in aging: Explaining the older person's life experiences.* Akron, Ohio: University of Akron Press.

Brink, T. (1979). *Geriatric psychotherapy.* New York: *Human Sciences.*

Brody, S. (1973). Comprehensive health care of the elderly: An analysis. *The Gerontologist, 13,* 412–418.

Crook, T., & Cohn, G. (1981). *Physicians' handbook on psychotherapeutic drug use in the aged.* Mark Powley Associates, Inc.

deVries, H., & Adams, G. (1972). Electromyography comparison of single doses of exercise and meprobamate as to effects on muscular relaxation. *American Journal of Physical Medicine, 51,* 130–141.

Danish, S., & Augelli, A. (1980). Promoting competence and enhancing development through life development intervention. In L. Bond & J. Rosen (Eds.), *Primary prevention of psychopathology.* Hanover, NH: University Press of New England.

Erickson, R. (1975). Outcome studies in mental hospitals: A review. *Psychological Bulletin, 82,* 519–540.

Flannigan, J. (1978). A research approach to improving our quality of life. *American Psychologist, 33,* 138–47.

Goldfried, M., & Davison, G. (1976). *Clinical behavior therapy.* New York: Holt, Rinehart and Winston.

Gotestam, K. (1980). Behavioral and dynamic psychiatry with the elderly. In J. Birren & R. Sloan (Eds.), *Handbook of mental health and aging.* Englewood Cliffs, NJ: Prentice Hall, pp. 775–805.

Hicks, R., Funkenstein, H., Davis, J., & Dysken, M. (1980). Geriatric psychopharmacology. In J. Birren & R. Sloan (Eds.), Handbook of mental health and aging. Englewood Cliffs, NJ: Prentice Hall, 745–774.

Hussian, R. (1981). *Geriatric psychology: A behavioral perspective.* New York: Van Nostrand, Reinhold.

Hyer, L., Barry, J., Tamkin, A., & McConatha, D. (1984). Coping in later life: an optimistic assessment. *Journal of Applied Gerontology, 3,* 82–96.

Jenk, M. (1984). Tardive dyskinesia: Special risk in the elderly. *Journal of the American Geriatric Society, 22,* 71–76.

Kalish, R. (1978). A little myth is a dangerous think: Research in the service of the dying. In C. Garfield (Ed.), *Psychosocial Care of the Dying.* New York: McGraw-Hill.

Lazarus, R. & DeLongis, A. (1983). Psychological stress and coping in aging. *American Psychologist, 38,* 245–254.

Levy, S., Derogatis, L., Gallagher, D., & Gatz, M. (1980). Interventions with older adults and the evaluation of outcome. In L. Poon (Ed.), *Aging in the 1980's.* Washington, DC: *American Psychological Association.*

Meyer, G. (1980). The new directions workshop for senior citizens. In S. Sargent (Ed.), *Nontraditional therapy and counseling with the aging.* New York: Springer.

Morgan, W., & Pollack, M. (1981). Physical activity and cardiovascular health: Psychological aspects. *Ergopsychology Lab Report, 26,* 1–15.

Neugarten, B. (1979). Time, age and the life cycle. *American Journal of Psychiatry, 136* (7), 887–894.

Neugarten, B. (1977). Personality and aging. In J. Birren & K. Schaie (Eds.), *Handbook of the psychology of aging*. New York: Van Nostrand, Reinhold, pp. 626–644.

Newsome, T. (1983). Symptoms of Alzheimer's Disease. Paper presented at the 36th annual Scientific Meeting of the Gerontological Society of America, Boston, Mass.

Penner, L., Eberly, D., & Patterson, R. (1983). Skills training for community living. In M. Smyer & M. Gatz (Eds.), *Health and aging*, Beverly Hills: Sage.

Poe, W., & Holloway, D. (1980). *Drugs and the aged*. New York: McGraw-Hill.

Powell, R. (1974). Psychological effects of exercise therapy upon institutionalized geriatric mental patients. *Journal of Gerontology, 29*, 157–161.

Schmucker, D. (1984). Drug disposition in the elderly: A review of the critical factors. *Journal of the American Geriatric Society*, 144–149.

Sparacino, J. (1979). Individual psychotherapy with the aged: A selected review. *International Journal of Aging and Human Development, 9*, 197–220.

Storandt, M. (1984). *Counseling and therapy with older adults*. Boston: Little, Brown and Company.

Veith, R. (1982). Depression in the elderly: Pharmacologic considerations in treatment. *Journal of the American Geriatric Society, 30*, 581–586.

Wellman, F., & McCormack, J. (1984). Counseling with older persons: A review of outcome research. *Counseling Psychologist, 12*, 81–96.

Whanger, A. (1980). Treatments within the institution. In E. Busse & D. Blazer (Eds.), *Handbook of Geriatric Psychiatry*. New York: Van Nostrand, Reinhold.

Willner, M. (1978). Individual psychotherapy with the depressed elderly outpatient: An overview. *Journal of the American Geriatric Society, 26*, 231–235.

Willner, M. (1978). Individual and group psychotherapy with the depressed geriatric patient: A rewarding approach. *Long Term Care and Health Services Administration Quarterly*, Winter, 308–332.

Wiswell, R. (1980). Relaxation, exercise and aging. In J. Birren & R. Sloan (Eds.), *Handbook of mental health and aging*. Englewood Cliffs, NJ: Prentice-Hall, 943–958.

Wolk, S., & Kurtz, J. (1975). Positive adjustments and involvement during aging and expectancy for internal control. *Journal of Consulting and Clinical Psychology, 43*, 173–178.

Wolk, S., & Tellen, S. Psychological and social correlates of life satisfaction as a function of residential constraint. *Journal of Gerontology, 31*, 89–98.

Zarit, S. (1980). Aging and mental disorders. *Psychological approaches to assessment and treatment*. New York: Free Press.

Self Medication as a Form of Self Control in an Intermediate Care Facility: Preliminary Data

Michael J. Salamon
Ruth A. Fulger
Salvatore LaVerde

ABSTRACT. This paper describes a project in which residents of an ICF were assessed on their ability to self-medicate. The goal of the project was to establish a sense of self control over some of their daily needs and thereby enhance well-being for those judged appropriate to administer their own medications. Sixty-four individuals (26% of the 249 residents) passed the three stage multidisciplinary screening process. At the end of the three month period, forty of the fifty-nine residents who chose to participate in the project were able to self-medicate, whereas nineteen were found to be non-compliant. Results to date indicate that a variety of issues need to be addressed before the true impact of such a project can be evaluated.

Over the years, theoreticians of human personality development have posited that most individuals have a strong motivation to gain a sense of control over their environment (Erickson, 1950, 1980; Piaget, 1952; Rodin, 1980). A sense of mastery seems to promote a healthier sense of well-being. In studies of situations where subjects are forced to give up their sense of mastery and control over their environment "learned

The authors are affiliated with The Hebrew Home for the Aged at Riverdale, 5901 Palisade Ave., Riverdale, NY 10471 in the following capacities: Michael J. Salamon, PhD is Research Division Director; Ruth A. Fulger, RN is Inservice Coordinator; and Salvatore LaVerde, PharmD is Director of Pharmacy Services. Please address inquiries to: Michael J. Salamon, PhD, 920 Broadway, Suite 1-A, Woodmere, NY 11598.

helplessness" occurs and reactive depression may develop (Seligman, 1975).

Institutionalization, particularly for the aged, has been linked with the theoretical position of losing control over one's environment (Krause, 1982). Being institutionalized requires an individual to adapt to a degree of regimentation rarely seen in one's home. Losing control over when to go to bed or wake up, when to eat and even what to eat are all part of the institutional life.

In a study designed to explore the sense of control over the environment and its effect on the general well-being of nursing home residents, Langer and Rodin (1976) manipulated the degree of responsibility individuals were asked to assume for plants which were placed in their rooms. Some patients were told that facility staff would care for the plants. Other patients were told that they would have to care for the plants themselves. At the completion of the study the researchers found that those patients who were given the responsibility to care for the plants were most alert to their environment and judged to be in better health than those who did not care for the plants. Follow up studies and studies with similar designs suggest that the heightened sense of well-being gained from developing a sense of mastery within an institutional setting endures for a significant amount of time (Rodin & Langer, 1977), and may even yield a reduction in mortality rates (Rodin, 1980).

Despite these optimistic findings, other investigators have suggested that an increase of personal control may not universally enhance one's sense of well-being (Janis & Rodin, 1980). This may be particularly true for aged individuals suffering from chronic physical ailments. Offering a sense of control to such individuals may be like offering the impossible and just add to the sense of frustration (Schulz & Hanusa, 1979).

Nevertheless, a variety of recent reports indicate that control over the environment can be given to institutionalized elderly albeit in limited directions. One of the more interesting areas in which attempts at providing residents of long-term care facilities control over their environment is in the area of medication. While policy in most states prevents patients in skilled nursing facilities from giving themselves their own medications, these policies frequently do not apply to the residents of intermediate care facilities in most states.

Conflicting reports exist regarding knowledge of medication and compliance among older adults. On the one hand, the aged were found not to be as accurate as a younger sample in identifying the purpose of the medications they were receiving (Klein et al., 1982). In a different study, the aged were found to accurately report the medication they were taking for severe or chronic ailments (Salamon, 1985).

The sheer amount of medication consumed by the elderly makes a self-medication program a potentially hazardous one (Harper, 1984). Given the proper supervision, however, encouraging residents of intermediate care facilities to assume responsibility for taking their own medications has been shown to promote a sense of control and independence, and strengthen the self-image (Madaio & Clarke, 1977). A self-medication program may also be an effective aid for assessing nursing outcomes and laboratory data (Meguerdichian, 1983).

THE PRESENT PROJECT

Recognizing both the possibility of a positive impact on residents' sense of mastery and control and the potential for abuse due to declining sensory abilities and increased use of medications, The Hebrew Home for the Aged at Riverdale undertook a new self medication program. This project was geared exclusively for the 249 intermediate care (ICF) residents who reside on six separate units.

A previous self-medication project at the Home was discontinued when it was found that residents were not compliant with their medication regimens. To overcome this deficiency, a rigorous preliminary evaluation of the residents' ability to accurately self-medicate was instituted. To insure proper selection of individuals to the program, all residents were asked to proceed through a three tiered assessment protocol. Though the procedure is rigorous it is non-threatening and not excessively lengthy. The assessments are performed by regular staff who are familiar with the residents. Unlike other projects where assessments for ability to self-medicate is done by medical staff exclusively (e.g., nurses, physicians, pharmacists) (Madaio & Clarke, 1977), assessments for this program are performed by a multidisicplinary staff. The purpose is to provide a more complete picture of the resident's level of functioning. First the unit social worker rates the resident on their mental status. This assessment includes an evaluation of the resident's judgement, levels of orientation, and alertness. Individuals found not completely alert or who are disoriented to time, place, or person could be assumed to also forget when to take their medications. If, however, they are found to be oriented they would then be asked to perform a variety of functional tasks related to self-administering medications, for an occupational therapist. The rationale for this stage of assessment is clear. If the patient does not have the necessary motor skills to put drops in their own eyes, keep count of their medications or open a (non-child proof) medicine bottle, they can not take their own medications.

The final assessment is performed by the resident's own nurse. This stage combines assessment with an educational component. The nurse instructed residents in why they take the medications they do, the dosage, times of administration and so forth. In order to be judged to be a viable candidate for the program, residents have to pass all three stages. A 30 day review is performed for assessment of compliance. If the resident is found to be consistently non-compliant by either having the wrong pill count or inappropriately taking the medication, they are counseled and eventually removed from the project.

FINDINGS TO DATE

As of the date of this report, the self-medication project has been in operation for just under six months. The first two and one half months were dedicated to the assessment of all ICF residents. Sixty-four individuals or 26% of the 249 residents passed the three stage screening process. Most of those individuals (90%) who failed the initial screening did so as a result of what was judged to be a limitation in cognitive abilities such that they could not be relied upon to accurately take their own medications.

Five residents passed the three stages of evaluation but refused to take part in the project. These individuals stated that they preferred not having the responsibility of self-administering their medications. Similarly, 29 residents, roughly 12% of the ICF population, refused to even be evaluated for the program. They too stated a preference for having their medications administered by their nurses.

During the second half of this pilot project, those residents who passed the three stage evaluation and wanted to self medicate were put on the program. Several of these individuals were found to be non-compliant. In most instances non-compliance was determined when it was found that residents had the wrong pill count at the end of the week. This signified that the residents were not taking the proper dosage of their medication. At the end of the three month period 19 of the original 59 individuals were found to be non-compliant and could not self-medicate. On the other hand, more than half, 40 of the original 59 were successful at self medicating.

DISCUSSION

While it is clearly premature to discuss the long term impact of a self-medication program on the sense of well-being for ICF residents this pilot data raises a variety of interesting and important issues not previously examined. While those on the self-medication project have to date, anecdotally expressed a better sense of well-being, almost 34% of the resident population of this particular facility stated that they preferred to have their nurse administer their medications. The majority of these individuals refused to even be evaluated for the project. Perhaps these residents recognized their own shortcomings and did not wish to be subjected to possible failure. Another possibility is that they may have become so institutionalized that they failed to understand the independence being offered them. Or, independence and control for them may have meant being able to tell the nurse to worry about giving them their medications so that they didn't have to. This would guarantee socialization and regular contact with the nurse.

The impact of passing the extensive professional assessment and then failing the requirements for remaining on the program is another issue to be examined. While the assessors all followed a relatively set criteria for selection to and removal from the program and the attrition rate does not appear to be significantly different by units, perhaps a personality variable is at work in the drop-out rate. Perhaps the assessors, wishing to promote independence and a sense of control, during the assessment overlooked certain deficiencies that would have precluded the resident's successful candidacy in the program. If this is the case, being chosen for a program despite certain deficiencies, such as this, and then being removed, may be viewed as a further insult to the residents sense of control and mastery. A further issue relates to the policy which implies that self-medication signifies an all-or-nothing ability. Perhaps, if it is found to increase well-being, individuals who would be found unable to self-medicate under the present guidelines when re-evaluated may be found to have the ability to self-medicate certain types or forms of drugs.

One conclusion seems reasonable based on our knowledge to date. While self-medication may be an effective way to promote a sense of control and thereby promote well-being for some residents the way individuals are selected for participation, their motivation for taking part in the program, and the impact of failure all must be accounted for before any conclusions can be made.

REFERENCES

Deci, E.C. (1980) *The Psychology of Self Determination.* Lexington, Mass., D.C. Heath.

Erickson, E. (1950) *Childhood and Society.* New York, Norton.

Harper, D.C. (1984) Application of Orem's Theoretical constructs to self-care medication behaviors in the elderly. *Advances in Nursing Science,* 29–46.

Janis, I.L., & Rodin, J. (1979) Attribution, control and decision making: Social psychology and health care. In Stone, G.F., Cohen, F., & Adler, N.E. (Ed's.) *Health Psychology.* San Francisco, Jossey-Bass, 487–522.

Klein, L.E., German, P.S., McPhee, S.J., C.R., & Levine, D.M. (1982) Aging and its relation to health knowledge and medication compliance. *The Gerontologist,* 22, 384–387.

Krause, D.R. (1982) *Home Bittersweet Home: Old Age Institutions in America.* Springfield, Ill., Charles C. Thomas.

Langer, E.J., & Rodin, J. (1976) The effects of choice and enhanced personal responsibility for the aged: A field experiment in an institutional setting. *Journal of Personality and Social Psychology,* 34, 191–198.

Madaio, A., & Clarke, T.R. (1977) Benefits of a self-medication program in a long-term care facility. *Hospital Pharmacy,* 12, 72–75.

Meguerdichian, D. (1983) Improving self-medication in an HRF. *Geriatric Nursing*, 30–39.

Piaget, J. (1952) *The Origin of Intelligence in Children*. New York, International Universities Press.

Rodin, J. & Langer, E.J. (1977) Long term effects of a control-relevant intervention with the institutionalized aged. *Journal of Personality and Social Psychology, 35*, 897–902.

Salamon, M.J. (1985) Medication use and illness: The relationship between self and provider report. *Clinical Gerontologist, 3*, 17–22.

Schulz, R., & Hanusa, B. (1979) Environmental influences on the effectiveness of control and competence—enhancing interventions. In Perlmutter, L.C., & Morty, R.A. (Ed's.) *Choice and Perceived Control*. Hillsdale, N.J., Lawrence Erlbaum Assoc.

Seligman, M.E. (1975) *Helplessness*. San Francisco, Freeman.

BOOK REVIEWS

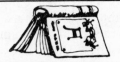

MEMORY FITNESS OVER 40. Robin West. *1985, Triad Publishing Company, 1110 NW 8th Ave., Gainsville, Florida 32601. 226 pp., $14.95, hardcover.*

Many middle-aged and older adults feel that their memory is not as sharp as it used to be. This book, written by a psychology professor who specializes in gerontology research, addresses the changes in memory associated with aging and provides strategies for minimizing their impact. The author contends that a good memory can be acquired through effort and practice. Just as physical exercise can keep a body fit, a daily memory work-out enables adult memories to function optimally.

The author cites several research studies in explaining what happens to memory as a person ages, but cautions that most of the tests utilized in investigating memory focus on lists of words or paired words. Such tests have limited relevance to daily life and do not actually focus on everyday memory. It is to the author's credit that this book emphasizes the practical aspects of memory research and application, rather than the more esoteric emphasis favored by the majority of academicians.

The chapter which deals with memory and self-concept emphasizes that a lack of self-confidence frequently prevents older people from maintaining or improving their memory. Such factors as anxiety, unrealistic expectations, a lack of effort, or lack of challenges can interfere with a person's realization of his or her full potential.

In another chapter, the author addresses memory and

health. She differentiates between the ordinary kind of memory lapse that can be avoided through the use of memory support techniques, and illness-related memory loss that stems from Alzheimer's disease, cerebral infarcts, and so on.

The second half of the book offers concrete suggestions on memory improvement. Special attention is given to remembering to take one's medication, remembering names, and improving attention span and concentration. A wide variety of strategies are discussed, including rote repetition, verbal elaboration, organization, and mental imagery.

This book is a clearly written and comprehensive introduction to memory and aging. Its strongest feature is the positive boost it offers by assuring the reader that it is indeed possible to enhance memory through the employment of simple internal and external strategies. While these strategies are not particularly unique or profound, they are practical and useful for people of any age. The book does not offer any in depth literature reviews, theories, or remediation techniques that professional readers might require, but professionals who work with middle-aged and older adults would be well-advised to recommend it to these clients and their families.

Ellen Lederman, MS, OTR
1518 Whitehall Drive, #203
Fort Lauderdale, FL 33324

DOWN MEMORY LANE. Beckie Karras. *1985, Circle Press, 11821 Idlewood Road, Wheaton, MD 20906. 156 pp., $11.95 plus $1.50 each, postage & handling. Maryland residents add 5% state tax ($.60).*

What started out as "light-hearted sessions for remembering the good old days" evolved into a very successful program enjoyed by a large group of senior citizens, according to the author. This book, written by a music therapist, is compiled of thirty-five (35) well-planned and adaptable programs for nursing home residents. Each chapter is a program in itself and is broken down into three sections: In The Mood; Activities; and Discussion.

In the Mood gives ideas for songs, music, and visual aids that relate to the theme of the chapter.

Activities includes ways that residents can participate themselves, i.e., watching short films, quiz questions, making simple craft projects, guest speakers, etc.

Discussion contains questions regarding the theme that are geared to resident reminiscing, and looking at today's issues.

What makes the book so useful is that the sessions are designed for a variety of functioning levels of residents. Some may be able to discuss, while other, more confused or non-verbal residents, can still enjoy the sensory-stimulation activities.

Each chapter theme was written to encourage reminiscing through such topics as: Childhood; Ice Cream Parlors; Big Bands; Hometowns; Old-Time Radio; Roaring Twenties; and Vacations. Each chapter contains sensory-awareness ideas, where to find resources, and some chapters close with ideas for refreshments that reflect the theme.

This book would be a worthwhile investment for the library of anyone responsible for programming for senior citizens!

Michelle R. Umbaugh
Activity Director/Music Therapist
Ft. Collins Good Samaritan Retirement Village
508 West Trilby Road
Ft. Collins, CO 80525-9989

WHAT'S NEW?

*INSTITUTIONAL CARE OF THE MENTALLY IM-
PAIRED ELDERLY*
Jacqueline Singer Edelson and Walter H. Lyons. 1985.
Van Nostrand Reinhold Company, Inc., 135 West 50th
Street, New York, NY 10020. 219 pp. plus Bibliography
and Index. Hardcover $27.95.

An important, easy to read contribution to the humane
treatment of the mentally impaired elderly! Sections include: (1) Individualizing Nursing Care; (2) Activity Programs; (3) Volunteers: L'Chaim—To Life; (4) Application, Assessment, Admission to Institutional Care and
the Role of the Family; (5) Institutional Challenges. The
sections of Activity Programs and Volunteers, are,
alone, worth the price of this book. Share this one with
all nursing home staff!

*AGING AND DEVELOPMENTAL DISABILITIES: IS-
SUES AND APPROACHES*
Editors: Matthew P. Janicki and Henryk M. Wisniewski.
1985. Paul H. Brookes Publishing Co., Post Office Box
10624, Baltimore, MD 21204. 446 pp. Hardcover $35.95.

The full scope of needs and services for developmentally disabled *older* persons are addressed in a collection
of writings by experts in this field. While this book does
not address Activities specifically, if the developmentally disabled are among your clients a greater understanding of their needs can be realized as they, too, are
aging.

INNOVATIVE PROGRAMMING FOR THE AGING & AGED MENTALLY RETARDED/DEVELOPMENTALLY DISABLED ADULT.

Paul M. Herrera, MEd. 1983. Exploration Series Press, P.O. Box 705, Akron, OH 44309. 187 pp. Soft cover $24.95.

I happened upon this book during 1985 and have found it invaluable! It is divided into three parts: (1) Nature and Need of the Aging and Aged Mentally Retarded; (II) A Model Program . . . Providing Comprehensive and Appropriate Programming; and (III) Implementing Innovative Programming—Strategies and Activities. Part III comprises the bulk of this book through the provision of Lesson Activity Sheets that include the Activity, Levels of Skills appropriateness, Objective, Procedure (detailed), Materials and Supplies, and Related Program Areas. Pre/Post Tests are included for measuring progress and Resources are listed. An excellent resource for meeting the needs of this special population that serves as a spring-board for additional activities.

Phyllis M. Foster, Editor

DATE DUE